Scars, Adhesions
and the
Biotensegral Body

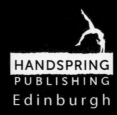

HANDSPRING
PUBLISHING
Edinburgh

Scars, Adhesions and the Biotensegral Body

SCIENCE, ASSESSMENT AND TREATMENT

Editors

Jan E Trewartha and Sharon L Wheeler

Forewords
Robert Schleip
Carol M Davis

Chapter authors
Joanne Avison
Leonid Blyum
Graham Scarr
John Sharkey

With contributions from
Wojciech Cackowski
Niall Galloway
Tracey Kiernan
Katerina Steventon

HANDSPRING PUBLISHING LIMITED
The Old Manse, Fountainhall,
Pencaitland, East Lothian
EH34 5EY, Scotland
Tel: +44 1875 341 859
Website: www.handspringpublishing.com

First published 2020 in the United Kingdom by Handspring Publishing
Reprinted 2020
3

ISBN 978-1-912085-46-0
ISBN (Kindle eBook) 978-1-912085-47-7

British Library Cataloging in Publication Data
A catalogue record for this book is available from the British Library

Library of Congress Cataloging in Publication Data
A catalog record for this book is available from the Library of Congress

Notice
Neither the Publisher nor the Authors assume any responsibility for any loss or injury and/or damage
to persons or property arising out of or relating to any use of the material contained in this book. It is the
responsibility of the treating practitioner, relying on independent expertise and knowledge of the patient,
to determine the best treatment and method of application for the patient.

All reasonable efforts have been made to obtain copyright clearance for illustrations in the book for which
the authors or publishers do not own the rights. If you believe that one of your illustrations has been used
without such clearance please contact the publishers and we will ensure that appropriate credit is given in
the next reprint.

Commissioning Editor Sarena Wolfaard
Project Manager Morven Dean
Copy Editor Dylan Hamilton
Designer Bruce Hogarth
Indexer Aptara, India
Typesetter DSM Soft, India
Printer CPI Group (UK) Ltd, Croydon CR0 4YY

The
Publisher's
policy is to use
paper manufactured
from sustainable forests

CONTENTS

FOREWORD *by Robert Schleip*

Wound healing is a fascinating process. It involves a dynamic interplay between migration, proliferation and differentiation of different cell types, the expression of cytokines and growth hormones, the synthesis and remodeling of extracellular matrix elements, and many other complex interactions. For connective tissue researchers like myself, one of the most intriguing facts in this colorful puzzle is the observation that during early human fetal development, wound healing tends to result in a scarless and complete regeneration of the original tissue, similar to the healing dynamics in so-called "primitive life forms", such as in an octopus that can regrow a lost arm. In contrast, wound healing in adult humans happens via repair, instead of regeneration, in which the original tissue is replaced by a different material than before and some kind of scar formation is usually left behind. These scars tend to impede the optimal functioning not only of the local organ, but also of the whole organism for a long time afterwards, and in many cases for the rest of our life.

What is it, that makes wound healing so perfect in an octopus, and in early human fetal development, and which we adults seem to have lost in most of our injury repair in everyday life? Wouldn't it be great if we could find some of the keys for evoking a more regenerative rather than reparative healing process? Wouldn't it be tremendously valuable for us to learn how we could influence the leftovers from previous injuries, in the form of imperfectly repaired scarring dysfunctions, and to complement the halted healing process with a more complete regeneration of the original tissue form and function?

If one studies the related literature on the potency of manual or movement therapy approaches in this respect, the scientific evidence tends to be rather sobering. Yes, with some very fresh tissue adhesions – such as in the abdominal cavity or in the superficial fascia – several forms of manual therapy as well as gentle stretching have demonstrated some beneficial effects. However, once the proliferative tissue repair phase has been completed, all attempted interventions which have been documented so far, have only shown minimal or no effects on the restoration of tissue architecture.

I vividly remember my excitement when I watched Sharon Wheeler for the first time working with decades-old dermal scars on human patients in a workshop she and I taught together several years ago. Was I hallucinating? Or was it true, that I observed the skin, after several minutes of gentle and skillful manual treatment, taking on a healthier color and texture than before? Not only that, when I examined the qualities of the tissue underneath the skin with my own hands, such as its adhesiveness, shearing mobility, and elastic properties, I could clearly feel a difference to before. For many clinicians this may be a nice re-confirmation of our common belief in the healing power of human touch. However, for the scientist in me this constituted a serious and troubling challenge. While the subjective impression of my eyes and hands (as well as of those around me) could be distorted by expectations and wishful thinking, would it be possible to examine some of these effects with more objective scientific investigations?

It is yet too early to report the outcome of our related ongoing investigation. However, some of my own spontaneous assessments of Sharon's work during a subsequent workshop, have so far been very encouraging. Whether with ultrasound imaging or a with a portable stiffness measuring device, I could observe a softening effect of the former scar tissues as well as a larger area around it. Needless to say, this demands more systematic evaluation in a properly controlled study. And what a blessing that Sharon is actively and vividly supporting such more critical evaluation attempts from her side as well.

Sharon Wheeler is a gem in the world of connective tissue manipulation and in wound healing. Her background in different forms of fascia-related therapies and her extensive experience in working with many thousands of patients and their scars is truly impressive. In this book she is complemented and assisted by Jan Trewartha, a well-known fascia therapist and a pioneer in fostering related interdisciplinary collaborations, in bringing this unique treatment approach for the first time to a wider audience.

While the influence of Sharon's novel manual therapy approach to wound healing is exciting enough, this book looks at the body and the effect of scars also from a biotensegral perspective. Biotensegrity offers a three-dimensional viewpoint of our human form, one that recognizes the constant adaptive interplay between the body and both internal and external forces, through the medium of fascia. Graham Scarr contributes a chapter on modeling the effect of scarring on this biotensegral interplay. Joanne Avison offers us an incisive introduction and an exploration of movement as affected by scars. John Sharkey contributes a dissection-informed discussion and Leonid Blyum makes the case for the counter-intuitive power of light touch work; this book covers such a wide range of topics.

Jan Trewartha's fascination for all things fascial has been expressed in her founding of the British Fascia Symposium, of which I am an enthusiastic supporter. I am very pleased to support her, with Sharon Wheeler, in this next project; the result is one which promises to deeply enhance the therapist's understanding of scarring, the effect on the body, and how to work appropriately to help resolve the (t)issues.

Robert Schleip, PhD, MA
Director, Fascia Research Group
Ulm University, Germany
January 2020

FOREWORD *by Carol M Davis*

We are not, inside, who we were taught that we were. As manual therapists and movement clinicians and teachers, we were taught an incomplete and downright erroneous view of human form and function. As technology, curiosity and a driving desire to get it right have advanced, a whole new 4- or 5-dimensional picture is emerging. This book educates us more completely and accurately as to the nature of the inner architecture and function of human beings, how that dynamic milieu is forever interrupted when scars and adhesions form to close the gap of injury and trauma, and how we can sensitively work with our hands, our hearts and movement to help restore inner symmetry and homeodynamic flow.

The energy of creation itself pulses through us every millisecond from the moment we are conceived. The standard two-dimensional linear textbook picture we studied that was "us", composed of separate hierarchical systems of solid-state matter frozen for our examination, has yielded to a living, multi-state, swirling, spiral, pulsing oneness of soft matter gel. Think about that for a second. No empty spaces, no layers, just a continuous dynamic web of soft matter matrix and cells from the top of our heads to the bottom of our feet.

No longer can we perceive fascia as "plastic wrap" surrounding all our muscles and organs. Every one of our 35–75 trillion cells is embedded within this living, vibrating multidimensional, biotensegral, fascial web. No longer can we see fascia as the container of all our separate parts – our organs, nerves, blood vessels, cells. We now know, according to Sharkey, Levin, Guimberteau, Oschman, Grunwald and others, that we can no longer think of our inner selves as separated into various functional systems and categories. We must truly understand that the internal milieu of our extracellular matrix is a wholeness, a oneness. Sharkey maintains that fluid, sensing, and organizing goes on continuously within this dynamic framework: **not** with separate systems "fluiding", "sensing", and "organizing", but **one** system working in various ways all the time, inseparable in form or function, to help us continuously evolve moment to moment, and ensure homeostasis and flow (Sharkey 2019).

Then catastrophe strikes: a wound appears. The oneness of the dynamic web is forever altered, and the miraculous body-mind automatically shifts into self-healing mode, plugging the hole and covering the gap with what we learned of as children to be a scab. The marvelous, pulsing, dynamic symmetry of the biotensegrity whole is interrupted by a patch. A living patch, but a permanent break in the symmetry. Depending on the location of this scar, we may forget about it, or we may obsess about it such that it becomes a part of our understanding of who we are.

Highly experienced manual therapists Jan Trewartha and Sharon Wheeler take us on a journey to better understand what is happening under the skin when scars appear and seem to heal, or not. In truth, the entire biodynamic fascial web will never be the same, and often these scars become the nexus of interrupted flow and function. Movement is altered and adjusted; pain develops often far from the site of the original injury. The continuous tension-compression biotensegrous dynamic is forever interrupted in ways comprehensively detailed in this book by leading practitioners and scientists. Trewartha and Wheeler then, with case studies and illustrations, help us learn, in detail, how we might help restore fluidity and harmony to the biotensegrity balance.

This book should be carefully read by all manual and movement therapists. It is comprehensive in depth and breadth, and generous in leading us to a more skilled and informed approach to helping our patients heal physically and emotionally from scars and adhesions.

Reference

Sharkey, J. (2019) Introduction to Fasciategrity/ Module 3 Our Basic Code. eHealth Learning TV online course. November 2019.

Dr Carol M Davis, DPT, EdD, MS, FAPTA
Scarborough, Maine, USA
January 2020
Professor Emerita
University of Miami Miller
School of Medicine;
Myofascial release physical therapist
Integrated Physical Therapy and Wellness
North Miami, Florida, USA

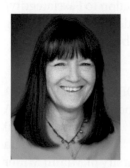

Jan Trewartha

Jan Trewartha (B.A. Hons.) is the founder and director of the British Fascia Symposium. She has been in healthcare since 1979, originally training as a State Registered Nurse in the Queen Alexandra Royal Army Nursing Corps (QARANC), working with patients on the wards and in the operating theatre; a superb (if non-deliberate) foundation for her future career. In 1988, being trained by a blind massage therapist to really feel the body, led to a lifetime passion for bodywork. Jan was a massage volunteer at the Auckland Commonwealth Games, where she learned from professionals of all modalities. Her work is the culmination of many years of training and experience in different disciplines. Through her school, Body in Harmony Training, Jan runs a variety of light touch therapy courses, including Sharon Wheeler's ScarWork, for which she was the first accredited tutor in the UK.

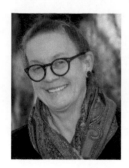

Sharon Wheeler

Sharon Wheeler's unconventional early schooling gave her a taste for the unusual. She found a welcome home in Esalen Institute's diverse educational community teaching Esalen's massage program in the 1960s. Deciding to take her fascination with the human body further, Sharon was fortunate enough to train with Dr Ida Rolf, PhD, in Structural Integration in the summer of 1970. Further training in Rolf Movement and Advanced Structural Integration in the 1970s consolidated her skills in this work, which she describes as "sheer joy to do." Her love of working with people and attempting the impossible, combined with a particular skill in sensing disruptions to the body's three-dimensional flow, have combined to generate Sharon's two discoveries: ScarWork and BoneWork. Sharon teaches these ground-breaking modalities in Continuing Education workshops around the world. She has a private practice in Structural Integration at her home in Port Orchard, Washington, USA.

Joanne Avison

Joanne Avison (MSS, KMI, CTK, C-IAYT, E-RYT500) is an author, advanced Yoga Teacher, Yoga Therapist and Structural Integration practitioner/teacher; she also has a master's degree in Spiritual Sciences. Joanne's fascination with fascia and human architecture led to membership of the Biotensegrity Interest Group, which pioneers how Biotensegrity distinguishes living movement and form. Joanne is passionate about the New Science of Body Architecture, the geometry of form and consciousness in animated beings. Her work includes writing the book *Yoga: Fascia, Anatomy and Movement* (Handspring, 2015) and presenting her ABC (Anatomy Basic Course) series worldwide, simplifying how fascia and Biotensegrity make sense of 21st century anatomy for manual and movement professionals of all disciplines. Biotensegrity is complex, yet it is also the keystone to natural motion and self-organized structure. Joanne's presentations weave the missing links between fascial anatomy and human health and performance, based in natural, biomotional integrity.

Leonid Blyum

Leonid Blyum (M.Sc. Cybernetics and Math at Novosibirsk State University and M.Sc. Clinical Kinesiology in Rehabilitation at Russian University of Peoples Friendship) is an internationally renowned physical rehabilitation specialist. His Advanced Biomechanical Rehabilitation approach is practised in more than 50 countries by caregivers and therapists of children affected by brain injury. He has been presenting at rehabilitation and bodywork conferences worldwide focusing on a better math = better therapy approach to hands-on practices. His first degree was in Mathematics and Cybernetics, later followed by studies and research in Kinesiology and Movement Analysis. This interdisciplinary perspective makes him a natural advocate of Biotensegrity as a powerful upgrade applicable to both traditional linearized biomechanics and organic empirical bodywork methods. Leonid is passionate about decrypting mathematically encrypted 21st century complexity sciences for practical use by bodyworkers and movement therapists.

Graham Scarr

Graham Scarr (CBiol, FRSB, FLS, DO) has a particular interest in the morphology and mechanics of living structures and has been at the forefront of Biotensegrity research for many years. He is a Chartered Biologist, a graduate in Microbiology, a retired osteopath, a Fellow of the Royal Society of Biology and a Fellow of the Linnean Society. He has produced 11 scientific publications and presents at meetings and conferences both in the UK and internationally.

John Sharkey

John Sharkey (MSc.) is an international educator, author and an authority in the areas of Clinical Anatomy, Exercise Science, human movement and the manual treatment of chronic pain. John is a graduate of the University of Dundee, the University of Liverpool and the University of Chester. He completed undergraduate and postgraduate studies in the areas of Exercise Physiology and Clinical Anatomy and he holds postgraduate qualifications in Education. He is currently a senior lecturer within the Faculty of Medicine, Dentistry and Life Sciences, University of Chester/National Training Centre, Dublin, and is the program leader of the Biotensegrity-focused, full-body, Thiel soft-fix cadaver dissection courses held at the Department of Anatomy and Human Identification, Dundee University.

Wojciech Cackowski

Wojciech Cackowski (PT and BCSI [Board Certified Structural Integrator]) has been fascinated with movement, sports and bodywork all of his life. He holds a degree in Sport Education and Physiotherapy, and he is also a structural integration practitioner and a teacher for Anatomy Trains. He has been practising manual and yoga therapy for the last 10 years and is the head of the Structural Rehabilitation Clinic in Ciechocinek, Poland. His fascination with fascial anatomy includes exploring spatial tissue relationships on cadavers, using ultrasound and analyzing movement, activities which have formed the basis of the Zoga Movement Project. Wojciech also teaches ScarWork as well as workshops that use Zoga and structural integration ideas in clinical applications.

Niall Galloway

Niall Galloway (M.D.) studied Medicine at Aberdeen University (1974) and is a Fellow of the Royal College of Surgeons of Edinburgh and England. In 1985, he was awarded the annual research medal of the British Association of Urological Surgeons for work on neurogenic bladder dysfunction. After fellowship training at Duke University, he joined the faculty at Emory University in Atlanta (1988). He is the cofounder and Medical Director of the Emory Continence Center (1992), a tertiary referral center for pelvic floor problems including prolapse and incontinence. He has worked in surgical reconstruction for urogenital anomalies and acquired defects of pelvic support anatomy, and in addition to clinical activities, he teaches Clinical Anatomy and has directed a medical school discovery elective in Human Symmetry. He has published on a wide variety of surgical topics, and his recent book, *Seeking Symmetry: Finding Patterns in Human Health*, explores nature's patterns in anatomy and disease.

Tracey Kiernan

Tracey Kiernan has almost 20 years of experience as a Dental Nurse combined with 20 years working as a therapist. She is the creator of Original TMJ Therapy®. Since first creating her unique protocol in 2000, Tracey has contributed to industry publications and books on her specialist subject and also to prestigious trade events as a speaker and workshop presenter. After traveling the UK and Europe as a teacher for over 15 years, in 2015 Tracey created her own training school, Blend Therapy Training. In 2015 she also co-created the unique Blend Fascial Facial® course, pioneering work focused on treating the fascia of the face. Her specialist knowledge in working with this area of the body also led to her oncology-specific Working With Head and Neck Cancer fascial training course in 2019.

Katerina Steventon

Dr Steventon (MSc. PhD.) is a skincare specialist with substantial experience of working at the clinical, commercial and research interface. She has an MSc in Clinical Biochemistry and a PhD in Transdermal Absorptions (phytoestrogens in postmenopausal skin). Having worked for Shiseido, La Prairie, Oriflame, Unilever, DSM, Merck and Smith & Nephew Wound Management, Katerina has an in-depth knowledge of skin science in both its healthy and diseased states, and a comprehensive understanding of the consumer perspective on facial skincare. She also runs an integrative private practice addressing clinical needs in acne, scarring, skin barrier dysfunction and skin aging. The principles of good practice in skincare form the basis of her clinical work as well as enhancing the well-being of her clients through self-care.

ACKNOWLEDGMENTS

This book would not exist were it not for the ground-breaking work of Dr Stephen Levin, who recognized the value of tensegrity as posited by Kenneth Snelson and Buckminster Fuller, and explained its relevance to the human body. Biotensegrity sheds light on previously ill-explained and outdated theories of human mechanics and further explains why restrictions in the body, including scars and adhesions, can have a globally detrimental effect, and why softening those restrictions can instigate a reversal of those effects. http://biotensegrityarchive.org/; http://biotensegrity.com/

The editors would like to thank the following people:
Graham Scarr for the generosity he has shown with his time, ability and knowledge as an editorial consultant.
All our expert chapter authors for sharing their skill and knowledge; without them this book would not have been possible.

All our other contributors who have added valuable insights stemming from their own particular fields of expertise.
Dr Katerina Steventon, Dr Sue Adstrum and Bella Reid for research support.
Adam Trewartha for photography advice and input.
All the "scar models" around the world who have helped ScarWork students develop their skills on the training courses.
Jeannie Kelley for her technological assistance with the online videos and her constant support.
Sharon Wheeler particularly wishes: "To honor my teacher, Dr Ida P. Rolf. The way she taught me Structural Integration as an 'artistic experiment' held the keys to the discovery of ScarWork. I want to thank my students and brilliant teachers for adopting ScarWork. Their contributions, support, and companionship mean the world to me."
Finally, the editorial staff of Handspring Publishing for their unfailing patience and support from start to finish.

How to access the online videos

Videos that accompany this book are available online: please visit wheelerfascialwork.com/library/videos or scan the QR link below.

The QR code can be scanned with a smartphone using an app, and many free apps are available to download. If you are using an iPad or iPhone running the latest software (iOS 11 or higher) then no additional app is required. Simply open your camera and point it at the code (no need to take a picture). A notification should pop down from the top – tap that and you will be taken to the videos.

FIGURE PERMISSIONS

Figures 2.1 & 2.2 © Fascia Research Society. Photography by Thomas Stephan.

Figure 3.3 Photograph reproduced by kind permission of Kevin C. Petersen, M.D.

Figure 3.5 Reproduced from Scarr, G. (2018). *Biotensegrity. The Structural Basis of Life* (2nd edition). Edinburgh, UK: Handspring Publishing.

Figure 4.1 Modified from Scarr, G. (2010). Simple geometry in complex organisms. *Journal of Bodywork and Movement Therapies.* 14(4):424–444. ©Elsevier.

Figure 4.4 (A&B) Reproduced courtesy of ©Theo Jansen. (C) Reproduced from Scarr, G. (2018). *Biotensegrity. The Structural Basis of Life* (2nd edition). Edinburgh, UK: Handspring Publishing. ©Handspring.

Figure 4.5 Redrawn from Levin, S. M., Lowell de Solórzano, S., and Scarr, G. (2017). The significance of closed kinematic chains to biological movement and dynamic stability. *Journal of Bodywork and Movement Therapies.* 21:664–672.

Figure 4.6 Reproduced from Guimberteau, J. C., and Armstrong, C. (2015). *Architecture of human living fascia: the extracellular matrix and cells revealed through endoscopy.* Edinburgh, UK: Handspring. ©Handspring.

Figure 5.3 Adapted from Wang, J. (2006). Mechanobiology of tendon. *Journal of Biomechanics.* 39:1563–1582.

Figure 5.4 Reproduced from Humphrey, J. D., Dufresne, E. R., and Schwartz, M. A. (2014). Mechanotransduction and extracellular matrix homeostasis. *Nature Reviews Molecular and Cell Biology.* 15:802–812.

Figures 6.6 & 6.10 Stecco, C., Sharkey, J., Schleip, R. (2018). Human Fascial Net Plastination Project.

Figures 7.1, 7.2, 7.4, 7.10, 7.11, 7.12, 7.13 Reproduced with kind permission from Art of Contemporary Yoga Ltd.

Figure 7.3 Images: by Joanne Avison; reproduced with kind permission from Art of Contemporary Yoga Ltd.

Figures 7.5 & 7.8 Reproduced with kind permission of www.mandukyayoga.com.

Figure 7.7 From *Interior Architectures*, Guimberteau J-C., (2009–2019). endovivo.com. Available at: http://www.endovivo.com/fr/architectures,interieur,dvd.php

Figures 8.2 and 8.3 Sheroes provides support and helps restore confidence. Photo credit: Hashim Ahmad Hakeem

Figure 8.4 The colourful Sheroes Hangout exudes a feeling of welcome. Photo credit: Hashim Ahmad Hakeem

Figure 8.5 Photograph reproduced by kind permission of Gilded Lily Design, paramedical body art clinic.

Figure 8.6 Photograph reproduced by kind permission of Yorkshire Mastectomy Tattoos.

As a State Registered Nurse in the early 1980s, I tended to have a rather linear image of the body, no doubt thanks to our textbooks which portrayed it, inevitably, in a dissected format. Handling patients was performed functionally, professionally, and was limited to giving them bedbaths, inserting catheters and taking blood, etc. This was all deliberately done in an impersonal way to maintain their dignity and it was considered inappropriate to touch them in any other way.

It was not until I trained in massage and developed a real sense of feel with my hands that I started to experience the body's three-dimensional connectivity. Therapists tend to develop an awareness of the inter-relationships between the body's various parts. For example, as we work on the head, clients may say they can feel "something happening" in the feet, or vice versa. When we experience this, we start to take tissue continuity for granted, but this is not necessarily a view shared by everyone. Like most therapists, I instinctively understood what I was feeling, and decades later the work of Dr Stephen Levin, in the form of biotensegrity, validated that intuitive understanding with science (Levin, 2006, 2019).

As a therapist, one of the hardest things to deal with is the frustration of not being able to help someone towards a better state of health. Obviously it is a two-way process; we are not just there to "fix" someone but to be a catalyst for them on their journey to well-being. Some people will never achieve this and there may be a number of reasons why not, but the majority of people will show at least some improvement.

However, when we do not manage to effect significant change then we must look at what else is going on. It is worth recognizing that adhesions may be affecting the internal architecture so much that it is not possible to restore balance until they are addressed.

When training as a nurse, I was taught that fascia acted merely as a protective layer which allowed structures to glide over each other; this was the extent of our knowledge at that time. Now the many roles of fascia are becoming better understood, with the popularity of the Fascia Research Congress (FRC), Fascia Research Society (FRS), and British Fascia Symposium (BFS) indicative of the high level of current interest.

In 2012, looking for someone to help me with a problematic scar of my own, I met Sharon Wheeler, and was so excited by the results of the treatment that I flew to the USA to work with her. I did not truly understand the relevance of scars and adhesions until I met Sharon; now I look at scars as a priority. Lower back pain? Check for C-section, inguinal hernia or hip/knee replacement scars as possible contributors. Neck or shoulder pain? What about the effect of that thyroidectomy, or even of that small chin scar from a childhood fall? Even tiny scars can have a surprising effect on the surrounding connective tissue, not just at the injury/surgery site (Chapter 10, p. 138).

Looking at scars in this way, combined with insights from studying biotensegrity, changes how one sees the body. Dissection courses are also invaluable, particularly those which are biotensegrity-informed, where the connections are tangible and demonstrable. An understanding of biotensegrity is vital to a hands-on therapist; it explains why the pain sometimes occurs away from the site of injury, and why when you treat one part of the body another responds.

In general, there is little public awareness of the damage that scars and adhesions could be doing to the body. The options offered by the medical system are few and range from "knuckling" the scar in an attempt to "break down" the adhesions, to surgical revision. There are many social media groups where people suffering from the effects of adhesions try to support each other; some of the stories are truly heart-rending. As this kind of therapy becomes more accepted, we trust that one day it will be standard postoperative treatment.

This book came from a desire to share what I had learned about working with scars over the years. Chatting one day to Joanne Avison, she suggested taking a biotensegrity approach. That germ of an idea developed into this collaborative book, in which many experts have written from their own perspective on the subject of scarring. I am grateful to them all for sharing their knowledge.

Bibliography

Levin, S. M. (2006). Tensegrity: the new biomechanics. In: Hutson, M., and Ellis, R. (editors). *Textbook of Musculoskeletal Medicine*, pp. 69–80. Oxford, UK: Oxford University Press.

Levin, S. M. (2019). Available at: http://www.biotensegrityarchive.org [accessed 19 August 2019].

Jan Trewartha
Windsor, UK
November 2019

Adhesiolysis surgery to remove or divide adhesions to restore normal function.

Anismus where the normal relaxation of the pelvic floor muscles fails during attempts to pass feces.

Arcuate line (line of Douglas) more formally referred to as the arcuate line of the abdomen. Also known as linea semicircularis which runs horizontally to demarcate the lower edge of the posterior layer of the rectus sheath. Scarring can be more common here as the inferior epigastric vessels perforate the rectus abdominis.

Atresia the closure or absence of any orifice or passage in the body.

Auxetic a structure or material that has a negative Poisson's ratio. It derives from the Greek word *auxetikos*, meaning "that which tends to increase", and refers to a tissue property that expands when lengthened. It is a particular property of human tissues.

Bleb a blister (often hemispherical) filled with serous fluid.

Chiral an image that is not superimposable on its mirror image.

CKC closed kinematic chain: the basic mechanics of tensegrity and living tissues.

Cytokines a category of signalling molecules that regulate immunity and inflammation.

Cytoskeleton the tensegrity organization of microfibers within each cell that regulates their function.

Davis's law relates to the growth of soft tissues in response to an imposed force.

Degloving one of the more devastating traumatic injury types where a significant portion of skin is torn away and evulsed or removed, similar to how one may slide a thin glove towards the distal tip of finger before removing the glove completely. Blood, nerve and lymph supply are totally severed.

Ecchymosis occurs when pooling of blood accumulates (i.e. hemorrhagic blotching) creating a hematoma more than 10mm in diameter. A discoloration occurs (i.e. bruising or purpura which are purple colored blood spots) just under or deep to the skin.

Exteroceptive relating to, being, or activated by stimuli received by an outside organism.

Fibroblasts a cell that synthesizes and maintains connective tissue, having an important role in wound healing.

Fulcrum the point around which two arms of a lever rotate.

Gastrografin enema a radiological examination of the colon and rectum by filling it with gastrografin, a water-soluble clear fluid that shows up on x-ray pictures. The examination is usually performed to assess if there is a leak outside the bowel.

Glycosaminoglycans (GAGs) a family of complex polysaccharides with important functions that include joint lubrication and maintaining the extracellular matrix environment.

Ground reaction force in biomechanical terminology, the ground reaction force (GRF) is the force exerted by the ground on a body in contact with it. It is exactly equal to the force of gravity upon the ground, as exerted by the body in contact with it. In other words, the weight thereof.

GLOSSARY

Heterarchy a multi-level organization where each part influences all the others in every direction.

Hierarchy a top-down organization where the top level influences all those below in a sequential way.

Hyaluronic acid (HA; conjugate base hyaluronate), also called hyaluronan, is an anionic, non-sulfated glycosaminoglycan. It is present throughout connective, epithelial, and neural tissues and the interstitium (Bonhams channels, prima vascular channels).

Hypermnesia abnormally vivid memory or recall.

Interstitium a virtual space between cells. The interstitial space is the primary source of lymph and is a major fluid series of tubes within tubes and their associated matrix present throughout the body.

Interoceptive relating to stimuli produced within the body, particularly in the viscera.

Keratinocytes responsible for forming tight junctions with the nerves of the skin. They also keep Langerhans cells of the epidermis and lymphocytes of the dermis in place.

Langer's lines topological lines drawn on a map of the human body. They correspond to the natural orientation of collagen fibers in the dermis, and are generally parallel to the orientation of the underlying muscle fibers. Using these lines for surgical incisions is recommended to reduce skin tension and allow for optimum scar healing.

Lateral raphe a ridge along the lateral margin of the erector spinae muscles formed by the aponeurosis of the latissimus dorsi, internal oblique and transversus abdominis muscles, and the layers of the thoracolumbar fascia.

Mobility referring to the ability to move, or to be moved, freely.

Muscle gaster the portion of a muscle located between the so-called origin and insertion is identified as the belly or gaster of the muscle. It mainly contains fascia and reddish muscle fibers with nerves, blood vessels and lymphatics.

Myofibroblasts cells that migrate to an injury site where they enhance the inflammatory response by producing cytokines.

Nociceptors "pain receptors", are sensory neurons that respond to damaging or potentially damaging stimuli by sending "possible threat" signals to the spinal cord and the brain.

Omnidirectional occurring in every direction.

Ontological relating to the philosophical study of the nature of being.

Pin-joint the simplified representation of a more complex (tensegrity) "joint" at a lower size-scale.

Proteoglycans complex hydrophilic molecules within the extracellular matrix.

Somatic memory memory of trauma stored in the body.

Stability referring to a state of being stable, implying firmness and solidity; the term is sometimes used to imply the opposite of mobility, for example, when a substance remains unchanged it is considered stable (as opposed to volatile).

Substance P a compound thought to be involved in the synaptic transmission of pain and other nerve impulses.

Syncretic an attempted fusion of different religions/philosophies/beliefs.

Tensile strength the tensile strength of a material is the maximum amount of tensile stress that it can take without breaking.

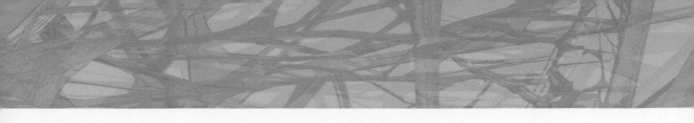

Tensional vector the direction where the tissue has the most tensional stiffness, or the strongest resistance when you push along it. The tensional vector is used to determine the working direction for applying counter pressure.

T-icosa the simplest omnidirectional tensegrity structure and the archetypal model for living tissues.

Toroidal the shape of or resembling a toroid. The most typical and commonly recognized toroid is a doughnut. In mathematics, a toroid is a surface of revolution with a hole in the middle (like a doughnut), forming a solid body. The axis of revolution passes through the hole and thus does not intersect the surface. The term "toroid" is also used to describe a toroidal polyhedron.

Trismus or Lockjaw, refers to reduced opening of the jaws caused by spasm of the muscles of mastication, or may generally refer to all causes of limited mouth opening or closing.

Wolff's law relates to the growth of bone in response to an imposed force.

Introduction
Joanne Avison

Chapter 1

"That nature applies common assembly rules is implied by the recurrence – at scales from the molecular to the macroscopic – of certain patterns, such as spirals, pentagons and triangulated forms. These patterns appear in structures ranging from highly regular crystals to relatively irregular proteins and in organisms as diverse as viruses, plankton and humans. After all, both organic and inorganic matter are made of the same building blocks: atoms of carbon, hydrogen, oxygen, nitrogen and phosphorus. The only difference is how the atoms are arranged in three-dimensional space."

Donald E. Ingber, The Architecture of Life,
Scientific American (Ingber 1998)

Biotensegrity can be (and has been) described as the key to understanding the structure of life (note the title of Graham Scarr's book: *Biotensegrity. The Structural Basis of Life*). Ingber's work (see the quote above and references within the book) in describing tensegrity as the founding organizational principle at the cellular, microscopic level is thoroughly researched (see www.biotensegrity.com), and therefore it is not a complete surprise that tensegrity structures can model movement and management of our living forms on the macro-level of the whole organism. Dr Stephen Levin coined the term "biotensegrity" to include and explain the living, structural and fluid dynamics of feeling, sensory creatures such as you and I, the "us" that strives to thrive rather than just survive as a whole living organism, reflecting the identical principles found at the microcellular level.

This book is about scar tissue and the logic of biotensegrity as a guiding foundation, or perspective through which to view and understand scar tissue as a matter of high priority in manual and movement therapy and practice. Jan Trewartha, Director of the British Fascia Symposium, as well as an ex-nurse and a practitioner with extensive experience, has been treating scar tissue as part of manual therapy, and has taken a keen interest in the importance of understanding the relevance of fascia to her work for many years. Recently, her time has been spent formalizing her clinical practice in this field, teaching and researching. The development of her own understanding of the relevance of biotensegrity to the effect of scars and adhesions led Jan to invite several of the world's leading protagonists in both biotensegrity and scar tissue treatment to contribute to this book, to help create a body of work which is set to become an invaluable resource for both current and future generations of practitioners.

Sharon Wheeler trained with Ida Rolf and has developed her approach to scar tissue over the last 40 years. Having originated Scar-Work and fine-tuned it over the years, she now teaches it to therapists around the world. Highly respected in her field, Sharon's focus is simply and consistently on disseminating her knowledge and deep understanding of transforming scar tissue.

"If the architecture of our fascial network is indeed such an important factor in musculoskeletal behavior, one is prompted to ask why this tissue has been overlooked for such a long time. There are several answers to this question. One aspect has to do with the development of new imaging and research tools, which now allow us to study this tissue in vivo. Another reason is the degree to which this tissue resists the classical method of anatomical research: that of splitting something into separate parts that can be counted and named. You can reasonably estimate the number of bones or muscles; yet any attempt to count the number of fasciae in the body will be futile. The fascial body is one large networking organ, with many bags and hundreds of rope-like local densifications, and thousands of pockets within pockets, all interconnected by sturdy septa as well as by looser connective tissue layers."

Robert Schleip, Foreword, *Fascial Manipulation: Practical Part* (Stecco & Stecco 2009)

Biotensegrity (see www.biotensegrity.com for further details), which has been researched extensively by Dr Stephen Levin, in particular from an orthopaedic viewpoint, offers a foundation to help explain movement and its restrictions in the variety of tissues Schleip refers to above. It is a model that also explains how those parts are presented in the living body, invariably as a whole. As complex a study as biotensegrity can be, it nevertheless simplifies a number of biomechanical issues by providing a universal explanation for the lasting integrity every organism maintains as a volume, throughout its life. Every living thing holds itself up in space, occupies its own volume and moves from speed to stillness, as a functioning, living structure. Be it a flower or a frog, a dragonfly or a Komodo dragon, a beast or a bird, a type of tree or a typical human being, we all share a structural ability to live on this planet as a whole, moving volume. Whether we move on land, in air or water, we all abide by the laws of soft matter physics in our elemental relationships to nature.

Biotensegrity defines how these rules are applied and expressed in animated forms, which is the keystone of this work. Jan Trewartha is primarily a practitioner. Like many who will pick up this book, she is devoted to making a difference to everyone who comes to her for treatment – invariably with a unique issue – but very often with something that the treatment of scar tissue can help. As practitioners with 20–40 years of experience, each of the contributors to this work can testify to a comment made by Jan Trewartha, that it is rare these days to meet anyone who is scar free. Scars can be a result of dental extractions or the process of giving birth, of growing up in a world where we routinely experience unexpected events that cause trauma to tissues, or caused by surgical interventions which could have been life-saving or routine. In Jan's world, scar tissue is to be expected, but becoming a victim of some of its commensurate issues may not be necessary. Jan's work at Body in Harmony specializes in (but is not limited to) scar tissue work, and it is from those experiences that her inspiration for this book arose.

In recent decades, during which fascia has been transformed from the Cinderella tissue of the locomotor system to the darling of many a therapist. Those of us versed in biotensegrity have found that a basic question we all ask in our various practices is: "Are there any scars?" The reason for this is obvious, once fascia is understood and appreciated in its many forms within the human body and especially in the context of biotensegrity. The role of fascia has only recently been fully recognized, despite the many pioneers who have argued for decades that fascia is a significant factor in many aspects of human health and performance. In this book, there is practical, palpatory guidance and background information for why it might be key to understand how scar tissue may contribute directly and indirectly to optimal movement. Thus, manual and movement practitioners across all disciplines may find their instinctive appreciation of what happens in life, in the field, on the track and in the movement classroom, and how scar tissue affects this, being reflected and supported by evidence in this book.

All of the contributors to this work have the grace and humility to acknowledge that we stand on the shoulders of giants such as D'Arcy Wentworth Thompson, Dr Ida Rolf, Kenneth Snelson, Buckminster Fuller and, among those more recently lost to our resources, Tom Flemons, each of whom made a remarkable contribution to the world of living structure and application that fascia and biotensegrity describe. We owe the latter term to Dr Stephen Levin, whose exceptional contribution to surgery, manual therapy and the lens through which this book is written, serves each of us writing here. We openly quote him, and have joined Jan Trewartha in producing this book to honor his huge contribution to promoting soft tissue intelligence and its remarkable applications to all movement, manual and medical therapeutic interventions. Our gratitude also goes to Donald Ingber for his work in the same field at the molecular level and to Robert Schleip for his service in reintroducing fascia to such an extent that it has now become part of our everyday vernacular. Our thanks also go to Jean-Claude Guimberteau and Jaap van der Wal for their contribution to integrating living tissues and embryological development pieces, for instigating the paradigm shift that biotensegrity is beginning to enjoy after 40 years of dedicated pioneering from Dr Levin, John Sharkey, Graham Scarr, Leonid Blyum and other protagonists. Sharon Wheeler, as Jan Trewartha's co-editor, trained in Structural Integration with Dr Ida Rolf in 1970. Like the other contributors to this book, Sharon's work is world-renowned for its appreciation of the multidimensional approach to the living body. As a Structural Integration practitioner, it was my pleasure to read Sharon Wheeler's contribution (Chapter 9) and to write this Introduction and also about scar tissue in

Chapter 1

movement (Chapter 7). Yoga is my personal favorite, as it offers the biotensegral basis of any movement practice and inspired the images which were taken especially for this work. As an early member of the Biotensegrity Interest Group (BIG, many of whom are contributors to this book), I have been part of a team dedicated to making sense of this emerging science, despite the range of misunderstandings to which it falls victim. Like many a new paradigm, biotensegrity is being gradually honed as it shifts our collective thinking from separate parts coming together ("contiguity", to use John Sharkey's term) to a state of connectivity in which we reveal our continuity, regardless of where we find ourselves. At all times, we remain whole and complete, from being zygotes onwards. Although all the contributors to this book have different specializations, each of us shares a sense of the living, multidimensional basis of the beings-in-bodies with which we work in practice.

This book is for all those who know, deep down, that there are no lines, no levers, no joints and no origins or insertions to announce the wholeness of the living body matrix – or any other non-linear biologic forms. Each of the protagonists featured here has helped carve the pioneering path that Jan Trewartha and Sharon Wheeler, as editors of this book, are taking. It is our privilege to walk and work with them, in the spirit of making a difference to the world. That benefit is not just for those individuals we treat, through the wisdom, theory, practice and examples illustrated in this book; it is also for those who read it, now and in the future, and feel a

profound sense of recognition, knowing that there is more to movement and manual therapy than intellectual and classical reasoning can bring (as valuable as such studies are in contributing to the complete picture). There are also instinctive and even intuitive aspects that resonate deeply with the spectrum of practical applications brought forth in this work. We need all three aspects of intellectual, instinctive and intuitive awareness. It is vital to have a resource that provides a reference to each aspect in a balanced way that honors how we actually work as practitioners.

There are still many who do not fully appreciate the wonders of our internal connective tissue matrix, the fascia. There are many more who do not grasp the nature of its wholeness, or why biotensegrity offers an explanation of how fascia works, one which has not been falsified in 40 years. Biomechanical principles of levers, and even linear principles of muscle meridians have been questioned; however, nobody has been able to falsify biotensegrity (assuming that they understand it, which few do). Many of the key protagonists in this field make contributions to this book, writing about both the principles and the theories they practice, providing application advice through examples from their clinics, so that their work is both informative and relevant to many different types of practitioners.

My prayer is that you will use this book thoughtfully and wisely, and that it will ignite your curiosity sufficiently to consider including its guidance in your own practice to promote intelligent, body-wide self-regulation for your clients. It will also encourage you to consider the advantages of gentle (low-threshold response) practices in both manual therapy and movement to promote well-being for both yourself and your clients. This is neither a method nor a list: it is a milestone on the path to excellence for anyone in bodywork.

May the most profound force-transmission system wisdom be with you. Enjoy.

Joanne S Avison

References

Ingber, D.E. (1998). The Architecture of Life. *Scientific American.* 278(1):48–57.

Schleip, R. (2009) Foreword. In: Stecco, L. and Stecco, C., *Fascial Manipulation: Practical Part.* English edition by Julie Ann Day. Padua, Italy: Piccin.

What lies beneath?

Jan Trewartha

Contribution from Niall Galloway

Looking under the skin

Fifteen years ago, I rarely heard the word fascia except in relation to houses, where it is used in the same sentences as the words "soffits" and "guttering". Training as nurses back in the 1990s, the extent of our knowledge was that fascia allowed structures to slide over each other and also protected them from damage. Now we read about fascia in the media, and the majority of therapists understand that it is a connective tissue of considerably more importance than was previously thought.

The Fascia Research Society and the Fascia Research Congress have been instrumental in the advancement of this understanding and, more recently, so has the British Fascia Symposium.

Fascia is, indeed, a type of connective tissue. There are other types, such as ligaments, tendons, bones, blood, fat and cartilage. The common saying is that "All fascia is connective tissue, but not all connective tissue is fascia", but the ongoing debate about what is and what is not fascia leaves this statement open to future revision.

Fascia is a generic word whose meaning has been linked to several different concepts: fascial (soft, fibrous connective) tissue, many fibrous body parts, as well as a complete, body-pervading fascial system. Unfortunately, these overlapping meanings have confused people's understanding of what fascia actually is. The international fascia research community has responded to this problem by developing two new terms: "a fascia" (Stecco and Schleip 2016) and "the fascial system" (Adstrum et al. 2017; Stecco et al. 2018), with the aim of clearly distinguishing between: 1) fascia; 2) fascial tissue; 3) a fascia (plural: fasciae) and 4) the fascial system. However, this definition is still evolving.

Fascia is a three-dimensional connective tissue comprised primarily of collagen and elastin fibers contained within a mucus-like ground substance of hydrated proteoglycans. The fibers within this extracellular matrix are largely produced by fibroblast cells, and its structure can assume many different forms according to its location and response to the forces imposed on it, that is, it is highly adaptive. Figures 2.1 and 2.2 show examples of this remarkable and adaptable substance which, in its different forms, outlines, envelops, pervades, blends and is continuous with virtually every structure within the body, right down to the cellular level. Physical forces can thus be transferred directly through the extracellular matrix to the cells contained within, which then alter their activity in

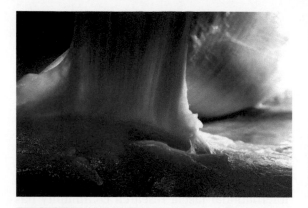

Figure 2.1

Fascia: a remarkable and adaptable substance.

© Fascia Research Society. Photography by Thomas Stephan.

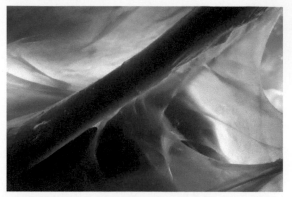

Figure 2.2

Fascia outlines, envelops, pervades, blends and is continuous with virtually every structure within the body, right down to the cellular level.

© Fascia Research Society. Photography by Thomas Stephan.

response and change the overall structure of the fascia (Ingber et al. 2014).

Different regions of fascia are often named according to their location, for example, the pericardium enfolds the heart, the pleura the lungs, and the epimysium sheaths a muscle.

Although Figure 2.3 shows the epimysium, perimysium and endomysium as separate entities, they are all structural variations of the same tissue with distinct mechanical properties. The endomysium transfers the force of myofiber contractions to the perimysium which, together with the epimysium, passes it on to the tendon and other connective tissues. The fascia is one structure, continuous and uninterrupted unless and until injury or scarring interfere with this continuity and, in doing so, disrupt the internal architecture and balance. Although the fascia can often appear as a network of two-dimensional layers that are peeled away during dissection, or revealed on an ultrasound scan, this description is misleading. All fascia is connected, even between the so-called layers, and it develops as a single tissue during embryological development. As Avison (2015) explains, the embryo unfolds, forming compartments and tubes that "all remain connected and continuous, although distinct and differentiated". The surgeon Jean-Claude Guimberteau also demonstrates this through his own investigations using high-definition endoscopy: "Contrary to conventional teaching, we now discover that there are no spaces, no separate layers of tissue sliding over each other" (Guimberteau and Armstrong 2015).

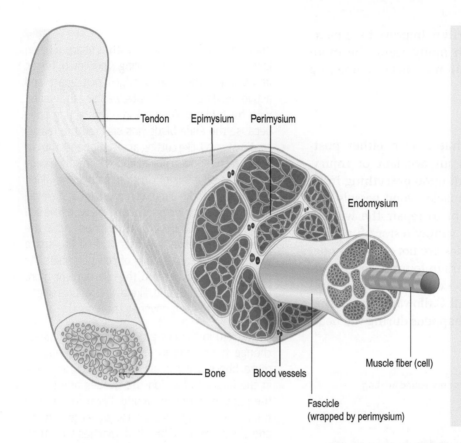

Tendon   Epimysium   Perimysium

Endomysium

Bone   Blood vessels

Muscle fiber (cell)

Fascicle
(wrapped by perimysium)

Figure 2.3
Schematic diagram demonstrating fascial continuities.

The fascia provides a continuous connective matrix, separating the body's compartments, both containing and connecting their internal structures. Schleip et al. (2012) characterize fascia as "fibrous collagenous tissues which are part of a body wide tensional force transmission system". It follows that a restriction of the free adaptive movement of the fascia will have consequences, to a greater or lesser degree, upon other body systems, regardless of distance from the original insult. Scars and the consequent adhesions fall into the category of insults to the body that can cause any amount of catastrophic damage, although the underlying mechanisms have not been well understood. However, with an understanding of the body's biotensegral architecture, the continuity of tissues and the complete enfolding of the body's structures by the fascia, the potential damage of adhesions to the body's function can be explored.

On the surface, a scar can look very neat and tidy. Sometimes the scar can be disfiguring, especially if it is on the face or somewhere equally visible, in which case the therapeutic aim would be primarily to improve its appearance. However, with many scars, the more important consideration is what is happening underneath the skin.

When the body has a scar, either post-operatively or from an accident or injury, the consequences fall upon everything in its path: skin, fascia, muscle, blood vessels and nerves. In its attempt to repair the wound, the body hastens to simply restore function; tidiness and aesthetics are not on its agenda. Wound healing occurs in four phases: bleeding, inflammation, cell proliferation and remodeling. See Niall Galloway's very visual description of what happens during the healing process (Box 2.1).

Box 2.1 Collagen fibers and wound healing
Niall Galloway

The fiber types and fiber density of fascia vary from one anatomical site to another, but the most common are elastins and collagens. Elastin fibers are thinner and are able to stretch to accommodate and recoil to restore form, but collagen fibers, although thicker, are not passive strands like dead straws in the mud mix of ground substance. Collagens are threads or strings laid down by fibroblasts, which are essentially fiber-making cells. The differentiation of fibroblasts into myofibroblasts or smooth muscle and fiber-making cells enables them to not only lay down these threads, but also to act as mini-winches.

Imagine slicing vegetables with a sharp kitchen knife and accidentally slicing your own finger. Immediately the wound edges pull apart and active bleeding floods the site, washing the wound with fresh blood. The wound edges spring open because the knife blade has severed the fascial continuity and, like cutting an elastic band, the cut edges recoil and are pulled apart. With the bleeding comes an influx of clotting factors and blood cells, and with the aid of compression and elevation, the bleeding will soon stop. The wound is still open, the cut is filled with clotted blood and, at the edges, myofibroblasts gather and fill the space with tiny strings consisting of collagen fibers. As more fibers are generated, the cells become more fixed in the tissues and, like a natural dressing, a scab begins to form, covering the wound.

Once fixed in the living tissues, myofibroblasts change their behavior, and instead of making more fibers, they begin to pull back and rein in the fibers to tension the tissues and bridge the gaps in the open wound. Local forces help the fibers to align as increasingly large bundles and sheets of myofibroblast winches with their collagen cables actively pull on the tissues and draw the wound edges together. Once filled with collagen fibers and attached to their mini-winches, the wound edges are drawn together until the scab is shed and the wound is closed.

This is nature's universal toolkit for healing any wound, a primordial process that has evolved over time.

The surgical wound is deliberately chosen, and for the best cosmetic results the surgeon uses Langer's lines when planning the skin incision,

continued

so that the scar will conform with the line of the collagen fibers in the skin. The skin is thoroughly cleaned and prepared before surgery to minimize the risk of infection. The surgeon is able to control the bleeding vessels and align the fascial layers, holding them in place with sutures at the time of wound closure.

On adhesions

Ideally the wound will heal in a manner that mimics the normal tissue alignment, so that continuity is complete, an apparently perfect match is restored, and the boundary of the old wound is virtually invisible. Commonly, an injury or surgical wound involves unavoidable tissue loss, and excessive tension or complications may arise, such as infection or necrosis of the wound edge that may leave a gap or defect too wide to be bridged by primary repair. Instead, a raw surface has to be left to heal, resulting in a shallow depression of wide scar that may lack the normal integrity and typical features of healthy skin such as pigmentation, hair follicles and sweat glands.

Some people have an over-exuberant reaction to tissue injury that leads to an exaggerated deposition of collagen fibers and thick wide scars called keloids, which may be very slow to soften.

Sometimes, in the course of healing, one fascial sheet will stick to another, causing adhesions that bridge a superficial to a deep "layer". For example, in a compound limb fracture, the periosteum of the bone may become fixed to the overlying skin, and the scar will be thin and hard (and often tender), tethered to the underlying bone. Small nerves are often severed in laceration injuries and, in the course of wound healing, regrowth may result in painful, bunched up bundles of knotted nerve endings in the scar called neuromas.

Some possible effects of scars and adhesions

Fascia, it is often cited, has a tensile strength of up to 2,000 lbs (~900 kg) per square inch (Katake 1961). This implies that a restriction in one part of the fascia, which will automatically be translated through the fascia, first locally, then distally, can potentially pull vertebrae and other joints into an unnatural relationship. In theory, a laminectomy scar might easily lead to misalignment of the spine, knees, pelvis or neck via the fascial continuities. A cesarean section could, for example, lead to problems with the hips, pelvis, back and/or knees. Can we envisage the likely path the restrictions and thus the effects will take? Not necessarily. In her 2005 paper, "Connective tissue: A body-wide signaling network?", Langevin summarizes: "Understanding the temporal and spatial dynamics of connective tissue bioelectrical, cellular and tissue plasticity responses, as well as their interactions with other tissues, may be key to understanding how pathological changes in one part of the body may cause a cascade of 'remote' effects in seemingly unrelated areas and organ systems."

It is well established that scar tissue can negatively inform complex molecular and cellular interactions while the body attempts to heal and recover (see Chapter 6). It is worth exploring the possible potential effects of scarring on different systems, as described below.

Chapter 2

The neuro-vascular tracts

In the One Series workshops, Sharkey and Avison (2015) stated: "The neuro-vascular tracts are all fascia all under tension and compression forces; communicating with each other through mechanoreceptors and mechanotransduction and the nature of their architecture. In other words, this body-wide signalling system doesn't simply send a nerve signal from nerve to nerve when one or another is plugged in... The connections are already there, and the means of connectivity is, itself, a sensory architecture; partly *because it is under tension*. Every tiny motion creates a resonance that is felt by the tissues, within and around the actual nerve. Rather than the specific nerve highways we are trained in, there is something more like a sensory hierarchy but one that can be manipulated." Again, "Nowhere is the tissue more dependent upon glide and elasticity than where the neural pathways, clothed in and invested throughout the fascia, map the microscopic pathways of the neural net." Thus, any minor disruption occurring due to adhesions could potentially affect any part of the neural net with currently unquantifiable results.

Keeney Smith and Ryan (2016) summarize Schleip (2003A, 2003B) in the particular context of scars: "Fascial restrictions (i.e. altered elasticity due to pathophysiological scarring) can exert an adverse effect on free nerve endings (functioning as mechanoreceptors), resulting in changes in tissue viscosity. This is particularly evident when the restricted fascia is challenged. Stretch or tensioning of restricted or dense fascia appears to trigger *incoherent* afferent signalling which in turn leads to aberrant firing sequences (i.e. muscle incoordination) along the myokinetic chain. Incoordination can lead to abnormal biomechanics, eventual abnormal muscle compensation and pain. 'Normal' fascial elasticity is essential for sound biomechanical and neurological functioning."

The meninges

It therefore makes sense to extrapolate that in such procedures as face lifts, scars are highly likely to affect the meninges via nerve sheaths that pass through the bony foramina into the skull.

Facial surgery or head injury may scar the periosteum of the skull (Figure 2.4). Think of the continuity: the meningeal tissues – dura, arachnoid and pia mater – are themselves specializations of fascia that line the inner surface of the skull, which is continuous

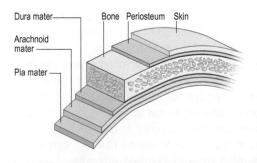

Figure 2.4
The fascial tissues associated with the skull.

with the skull periosteum. As the pia mater can scarcely be dissected from the brain and spinal cord, and the dura mater continues with the spinal nerves as they exit between the vertebrae, consider the possible consequences to the nervous system as a whole.

The cell

Jorgens et al. (2017) state that "Our finding of an intermediate filament cage surrounding the [cell] nucleus, and occasionally passing into the nuclear space through invaginations or tunnels in the nucleus, suggests a unique mechanical coupling between receptors on the plasma membrane and the nucleus that have not been found in previous work in mesenchymal-type cells cultured on rigid substrata." Mina Bissell, of the Lawrence Berkeley National Laboratory, commented: "The reason we're excited is that it explains a whole lot of literature of how force and tension could be playing a role together with biochemical signals to bring about huge changes in a cell" (Yang 2017). This research has interesting implications regarding the potential effect of adhesions, with the high probability that a compressed and restricted system creating abnormal force patterns could interfere with cellular function (Ingber et al. 2014).

Anything, therefore, which has caused a degeneration of soft tissue and reduced fascial elasticity can affect the severity of a scar's impact on the body (see Chapter 3, pp. 24–25). For example, a golfer who has spent 20 years swinging to the left when playing without attempting any corrective exercise or manual therapy, may have developed a rotation in the torso and possibly the pelvis. This could be the result of fibroblasts laying down extra collagen fibers along particular lines of tensional force, so that repetitive actions result in reinforcement and strengthening along these lines; this may limit mobility in other planes of movement. The rotation may then be translated into other parts of the body unless fascial bodywork is used to clear these holding patterns. An uneven distribution of force throughout the body will occur, and consequently some joints may take the strain of this more than others. We only have to look at the structural problems of our professional golfers and tennis players to see this process in action. If, for example, our golfer then undergoes a meniscus repair to rectify long-term damage to the knee, any adhesions may then link into other soft tissues which have degenerated through overuse. A scar can develop adhesions that extend deep into the subcutaneous tissues as the tensional forces within follow the lines of least resistance (see Chapter 4, Figure 4.7).

Looking at the continuities, Bordoni and Zaner (2013) stated: "Consideration should be given to the fascial system of the lower limbs, communicating with the whole body, and in particular with the thoracolumbar fascia. The gluteal fascia departs from the iliac crest and, through the sacrum and the coccygeal bone, runs to the femoral fascia; the latter will then become the tibial fascia, involving the tibia and fibula, finally enclosing the whole foot. The gluteus maximus is part of the thoracolumbar fascia, and the fascia of the lower limbs is its logical extension. We can then assume that if a scar on the ankle creates an adhesion, this unusual tension will also be recorded by the thoracolumbar fascia, with the consequent appearance of back pain or dysfunctions in the shoulders."

Full connectivity, via the fascia, was demonstrated to me on a biotensegrity-informed dissection course. On one cadaver, the left shoulder joint and the right foot were dissected down to the deep fascia. The shoulder, and then the foot, were moved in turn; whichever joint was moved, the other one could also be seen to move, showing the fascial connection that existed between them. Witnessing this with my own eyes proved, albeit empirically, that if these were mobile structures only limited in their movement by scarring, then the resultant restriction could be similarly passed through the tissues creating a distal reflection. It also invites the possibility that if scar tissue can be rendered more mobile through scar therapy, there may well be consequent restoration of function in the locally and distally impacted sites.

We have looked here at just some of the possible effects of scarring; in conclusion, the results of scars and adhesions might be devastating on a level that we cannot presently fully analyze.

Even small scars can be damaging

When we consider scars that will cause problems, we should also include small scars. Their effects may appear to be local although, as discussed later in this chapter, even the smallest scar may have further, invisible ramifications (Figures 2.5A,B and 2.6A,B).

A small, surgically induced scar that can have major consequences may be the result of keyhole surgery, which is an approach increasingly being used for operations that previously involved a linear incision. For example, in laparoscopies, the abdomen is inflated with gas and tools are introduced, including a light source. This is generally promoted as a minimally invasive technique, and indeed it is, in comparison to previous methods. However, the tracking adhesions that may develop can create their own problems, with extensive exploration of the abdomen causing damage wherever the surgeon's tools are used. Kavic et al. (2010) noted that in one review of open operations, 71% of adhesions involved the laparotomy scar, and that multiple laparotomies could increase the incidence of adhesions to as high as 93%. They summarized: "It seems that laparoscopy is not a panacea for the prevention of abdominal or pelvic adhesions. Like open surgery, minimally invasive surgery necessarily involves peritoneal and tissue trauma."

It is shocking, if fascinating, how an apparently simple, minimally disruptive operation can potentially cause further problems.

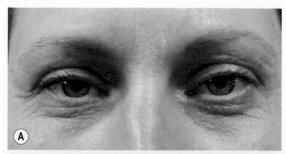
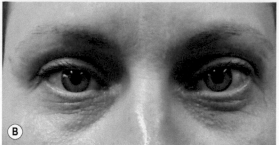

Figure 2.5A,B

(A) Pre-treatment; (B) post-treatment. Four small scars: (i) one lateral to the left eye since babyhood, origin unknown; (ii) one above the left eyelid from a fall, resutured when sutures were removed too early; (iii) one above the right eyelid, origin unknown; and (iv) one between the eyebrows. Note that (iii) and (iv) occurred as a result of an assault. All of the scars are very faint. The client reported: "My forehead immediately felt relaxed after the students worked on my scars, I couldn't believe the difference it made. As I was used to it always feeling tight, especially my brow line, I also noticed I didn't appear as if I was frowning or scowling as much." We can see that the right eye, in particular, is more open, with less loose tissue underneath.

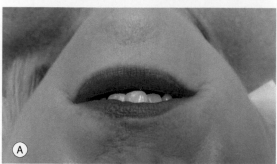
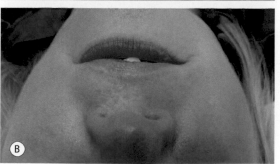

Figure 2.6A,B

Left unilateral cleft lip repair. (A) Pre-treatment; (B) post-treatment. Despite several surgical repairs, this client is still conscious of her scar. However: "ScarWork[1] has improved the scar immeasurably, without the need for more surgical intervention. I feel more engaged and accepting of my scar since receiving treatment, which is a real breakthrough for me." Here, we can see that the lips were, even at rest, apart, whereas now there is less tension and improved skin texture.

---

1   Where the term "ScarWork" is used, this refers to Sharon Wheeler's ScarWork. The term "scar therapy", when used, refers generally to any modality addressing scar tissue.

In each case, the manner in which adhesions affect the client is unique. Various elements can influence the path that adhesions take. Where there is another scar nearby the first, it has been noted by scar therapists that the adhered tissue from one scar appears to connect into the other.

Changing how scars are viewed

Recently, throughout the caring professions, awareness of the damage that scars can bring has increased. Surgeons, of course, are used to "revising" scars through further surgery, going back into the same scar and clearing the adhesions. However, in all probability, further adhesions may develop thereafter, so this is often only a temporary solution to the problem. Surgeons will also sometimes refuse to operate further because more adhesions are the inevitable result. These would further weaken tissue, reduce mobility and, years later, could be just as painful, and therefore, although this is a rational decision, the patient is left in limbo, and in pain, with nowhere to go.

Scar revision surgery – is it always necessary?

This woman (Figure 2.7A,B) had tendon surgery in her late teens, but when these photographs were taken in her 50s she could not remember the details. In two weeks' time she was scheduled for the removal of three of the distal toe phalanges as their position, turning under her foot, made walking painful.

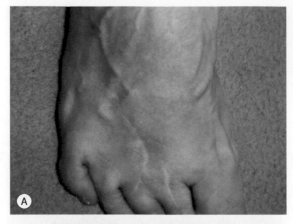

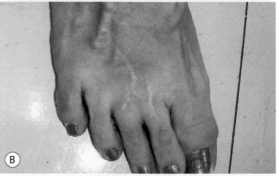

Figure 2.7
(A) Pre-treatment: distortion of what would once have probably been linear scars, and of the toes. (B) After two treatments. The toes are straighter resulting in a more normal foot shape.

Photography: Sarah Strong.

Figure 2.7A shows an informal photograph, taken for the record by the therapist. During two sessions, about a week apart, each lasting about 30–40 minutes, the foot was worked on with ScarWork; no other modality was employed. After a fortnight the client reported that her toes had straightened out

(Figure 2.7B) and subsequently she cancelled the planned operation.

It was thus concluded that the adhesions from the original scars had caused the deformation of the toes; by working on the scars and adhesions the soft tissues returned to a more acceptable shape and the toes to more normal alignment. It should be emphasized here that the client would then most probably have benefited from manual therapy to redress the severe compensation patterns that would have developed around the deformed foot over the decades.

An understanding of the power of adhesions to create such a deformity could inform many other potentially unnecessary surgical decisions and consequently save patients years of discomfort or pain.

Scars in therapy work

ScarWork appears to be effective in the majority of cases, regardless of whether a scar is old or new[2]. However, once the scar has been worked on, compensation patterns, as illustrated above (Figure 2.7AB), occurring during decades of adaptation to the problem that have caused the client possible discomfort or pain as well as a lack of mobility, ideally need to be addressed using one of the many fascia-focused modalities aimed at clearing these holding patterns.

---

2 ScarWork is not given until the client has been discharged by the surgeon. See Chapter 9 for contraindications.

Helping a client to return to their pre-operative body shape is impossible if they are internally torqued by scarring. The word realignment is often used; this is not an attempt to create perfect alignment in a client, but rather to restore them towards what was normal before the internal scarring distorted their body. Indeed, rebalancing may be a more appropriate word. We are all different and we celebrate those differences, but we demonstrate our histories in the way we stand, walk and hold ourselves. Although it is possible to assist clients with the results of many injuries, there may be some postural irregularities which will never clear, for whatever reason.

As the body is restored to a more normal alignment and the myofascial restrictions created by scars and adhesions soften, it is vital for integration to occur, facilitated by the therapist. Integration enables a physical and emotional reconnection of parts of the body that have previously felt disconnected from each other; for the client, this results in a sensation of restored wholeness (see Chapter 10).

How does understanding biotensegrity change how we see scars?

Our current knowledge of scars and adhesions gives sufferers hope and opens up a whole field of potential research into the possible effects of adhesions upon the different systems of the body. As a therapist, there is nothing more disheartening than being unable to help someone in pain, but when we see that the pain may stem from the compressive, distorting effects of adhesions and we know how to address those issues, there are grounds for optimism that working on the scars will provide at least some improvement in the client's condition.

The biotensegrity concept explains how living cells, tissues, organs and the entire body can be coupled into a complete functional unit, with each of its parts remaining stable at every moment of its existence. Any change in this arrangement caused by the formation of scars and adhesions will alter the normal balance of forces within the tissues and potentially lead to symptomatology. Our bodies are constantly remodeling themselves according to the stresses imposed upon them, and it is this particular organization of its multiscale anatomy which determines how these forces are distributed to the tissues and cells.

What happens to body architecture when scars are worked on?

We cannot get rid of scars and adhesions. The aim is to reintegrate the scar tissue into the three-dimensional fascial matrix by directly changing the tissue tension and enabling the system to reorganize itself. Scar therapies can change the appearance of scars and the way in which they influence the surrounding tissues, thus leading the client to report feelings of more freedom, mobility and improved sensory function (although more research is still needed to establish how these benefits are achieved).

On occasions scars can be advantageous and they become an integral part of the body, necessary for its adaptive functioning (see Chapter 3, pp. 30–31).

What is the potential of treating scars as standard practice?

If surgeons referred their patients for scar therapy once they had been discharged, what would be the consequences? To be fair, not every patient experiences pain or discomfort from their scars, but, as demonstrated, the results may be more insidious and not necessarily obvious. We cannot quantify precisely the possible effects of scarring or of using scar therapies, but the empirical evidence alone suggests that there would be potential improvement in the quality of life for clients, and lower costs because of fewer analgesics and anti-inflammatories, as well as a reduced need for scar revision surgery. Some hospitals in the UK are already trialing ScarWork, and pilot studies and further research are underway. These are exciting times.

References

Adstrum, S., Hedley, G., Schleip, R., Stecco, C., and Yucesoy, C. A. (2017). Defining the fascial system. *Journal of Bodywork and Movement Therapies.* 21:173–177.

Avison, J. S. (2015). *Yoga: Fascia, Anatomy and Movement* (1st edition). Edinburgh, UK: Handspring Publishing.

Bordoni, B., and Zaner, E. (2013). Skin, fascias and scars: symptoms and systemic connections. *Journal of Multidisciplinary Healthcare.* 7:11–24.

Guimberteau, J.-C., and Armstrong, C. (2015). *Architecture of Human Living Fascia.* Edinburgh, UK: Handspring Publishing.

Ingber, D. E., Wang, N., and Stamenović, D. (2014). Tensegrity, cellular biophysics and the mechanics of living systems. *Reports on Progress in Physics.* 77:046603.

Jorgens, D. M., Inman, J. L., Wojcik, M., Robertson, C., Palsdottir, H., Tsai, W.-T., Huang, H., Bruni-Cardoso, A., López, C. S., Bissell, M. J., Xu, K., and Auer, M. (2017). Deep nuclear invaginations are linked to cytoskeletal filaments – integrated bioimaging of epithelial cells in 3D culture. *Journal of Cell Science.* 130:177–189.

Katake, K. (1961). The strength for tension and bursting of human fasciae. *Journal of Kyoto Prefectural University of Medicine.* 69:484–488.

Kavic, M., Kavic, M., and Kavic, S. (2010). *Adhesions and Adhesiolysis. Prevention and management of laparoendoscopic surgical complications* (3rd edition). Society of Laparoendoscopic Surgeons. Available at: https://laparoscopy.blogs.com/prevention_management_3/2010/10/adhesions-and-adhesiolysis.html [accessed 20 November 2018].

Keeney Smith, N., and Ryan, C. (2016). *Traumatic Scar Tissue Management,* p. 73. Edinburgh, UK: Handspring Publishing.

Langevin, H. (2005). Connective tissue: A body-wide signaling network? *Medical Hypotheses.* 66:1074–1077.

Schleip, R. (2003A). Fascial plasticity – a new neurobiological explanation: Part 1. *Journal of Bodywork and Movement Therapies.* 7:11–19.

Schleip, R. (2003B). Fascial plasticity – a new neurobiological explanation: Part 2. *Journal of Bodywork and Movement Therapies.* 7:104–116.

Schleip, R., Findley, T., Chaitow, L., and Huijing, P. (2012). *Fascia, the tensional network of the human body.* Edinburgh, UK: Churchill Livingstone Elsevier.

Sharkey, J., and Avison, J. S. (2015). The One Series workshops: *One Nerve.* North London School of Sports Massage, London, UK. 17 November 2015.

Stecco, C., Adstrum, S., Hedley, G., Schleip, R., and Yucesoy, A. (2018). Update on fascial nomenclature. *Journal of Bodywork and Movement Therapies.* 22:354.

Stecco, C., and Schleip, R. (2016). A fascia and the fascial system. *Journal of Bodywork and Movement Therapies.* 20:139–140.

Yang, S. (2017). The strings that bind us: cytofilaments connect cell nucleus to extracellular microenvironment. Available at: https://phys.org/news/2017-01-cytofilaments-cell-nucleus-extracellular-microenvironment.html [accessed 4 November 2018].

The adaptive body

Jan Trewartha

Contributions from Niall Galloway and Tracey Kiernan

Tissue goes home

Having trained in ScarWork[1], I found that my understanding of the body became even more three-dimensional: experiencing at a deeper level practical application of the mantra "tissue will always go home" with tangible proof that light touch is effective (see Chapter 5), compounded by the realization that tissue responds no matter how old a scar is, were lightbulb moments for me. Understanding these factors helps a therapist to respect the body's ability to self-heal; we are only catalysts, after all, as much as our egos would like us to be the wavers of magic wands. The gentle touch, knowing when to stop, trusting the tissue to respond – these really do make light work of helping the body to restore itself to health.

What I did not fully understand before working with scars is the way in which tissue can be moved, or rather, how it can be facilitated so that it "goes home". Imagine a dog bite that has lifted a V-shaped piece of skin and its underlying tissue, which are then sewn back into place in the Accident and Emergency department. It may be a good suturing job, yet if you were to examine the area under a microscope you would see the slight displacement that results from attempting to reassemble the complexity of human tissue; this can be likened to trying to complete an intricate, three-dimensional jigsaw puzzle. Imagine that, as a therapist, you could pin the displaced tissue down firmly but gently, drop into it and follow it as it moves fractionally, rotating and angling, until it repositions itself correctly. It feels as though the three-dimensional puzzle is clicking into place, followed by a pulsing and a relaxation of the tissue. Next, look at the tissue again and see how much better it sits, how much more integrated the surrounding tissues feel, and how naturally plumped up they have become as the fluids flow more easily through the area.

Similarly, a cesarean section (C-section) may leave a woman with her *mons pubis* slumped, losing the curvature that is a part of her natural shape. Retractors used during surgery leave a retraction pattern that can prevent tissue from settling back into its former position. Furthermore, as the surgeon Niall Galloway (2018) explains: "Lymphatic drainage is from the mons to the groins and a transverse scar or scars may embarrass lymphatic drainage." Emergency C-sections are most likely to generate a slumped *mons pubis*; and, as Galloway (2018) clarifies: "In a transverse wound the key layer is called

---

1   Where the term "ScarWork" is used, this refers to Sharon Wheeler's ScarWork. The term "scar therapy", when used, refers generally to any modality addressing scar tissue.

Scarpa's fascia. It lies between two fatty layers between the rectus fascia – the thick leathery layer immediately covering the rectus abdominis muscles – and the skin. In a C-section, the rush is to safely deliver this baby and then hurry up to deliver the next who might be waiting in the wings. Unlike typical elective surgery the obstetricians often have to rush the closure and fail to repair Scarpa's fascia. This makes all the difference to how and whether the wound will heal properly." Displaced tissues can often be encouraged to "go home"; that is, once scar therapy has helped to restore the fascial integrity, it is often possible to help the *mons pubis* return to its normal position, with the client then recovering some or all of her female shape and a feeling of deep, inner connectivity.

Changing how we view the body

It doesn't seem possible that the body should respond so easily and readily to light touch applied in the correct way, but it does (Chapter 5). Understanding the most important factor here, that a therapist's role is to enable the natural self-healing of the body, to not force it or be heavy-handed with it, can transform our practice. Add to that a comprehension of the body's biotensegral nature and we grasp that when one piece of tissue is displaced (for whatever reason), not only is the integration of tissue affected proximally but, via the fascial continuities, may translate to more distal tissues. This must affect fluid flow and functionality – How could it not? It is this understanding of the three-dimensional continuity of structures and the resulting ordered distribution of force throughout the body that shifts our view of the body paradigm and should potentially impact radically and beneficially upon the traditional medical approach to patient care.

Balance and integrity of structure

Our bodies are naturally designed to be energy-efficient and in balance, and biotensegrity explains how they can operate as minimal energy systems, in which minimum effort = maximum efficiency. However, at any time during our lives, there are many ways in which simple ease of movement and efficient energy use can be compromised.

As we grow up, we frequently injure ourselves, undergo operations, develop infections or inflammatory diseases that create internal scarring, and/or acquire daily behavioral patterns which may affect our posture. In this way, mobility can be compromised, discomfort or pain can develop, and thus each of our bodies has to adapt to the demands which we place upon it – we call this "compensation". Energy levels can be lowered, our mobility reduces, and we can find ourselves slowing down. We are versatile creatures and therefore it only takes a short time for us to accept the new paradigm, even if it is more restrictive, and then adapt to a new way of being and feeling. Self-awareness (and some are more self-aware than others) alerts us to these sometimes minute changes and their accumulation over subsequent months then years and, if we are active, we are more likely to register those changes. The older, less active, very busy or unaware person may not comprehend that something has altered within them, and may attribute any discomfort, stiffness, swelling and/or reduced mobility to advanced age, overworking or being stressed. By the time the individual realizes what is happening the effects have accumulated, resulting in more serious limitations. However, it does not necessarily have to end up this way; indeed, an understanding of the body's dynamics can inform how we care for ourselves and our clients.

Comprehending that bodies are self-contained organisms, "compliant and flexible structures that are highly resilient to the effects of external forces" (Scarr 2018, page 137), enables us to view them differently. We can see that when compromised by any of the disruptive effects of repetitive strain patterns, for example, injuries, the compliant and flexible body will adapt.

Fourie and Sharkey (2018) point out that inserting a foreign object into the body, as in a hip replacement, disrupts the continuity of the tissues. Yet the biotensegral body will always adapt to any change and carry on because the underlying principles of tissue organization remain the same: adaptations may not be comfortable, and may even result in pain, but the body will always try to maintain functionality in the most efficient and best way possible; it is an inherent survival strategy. Scarr (2018, page 137)

states: "A tensegrity configuration automatically balances itself, creates a highly efficient control strategy that is built into the structure itself and contributes to dynamic stability."

The way in which invisible forces are disseminated throughout the body will always alter around an injury (see Chapter 4, Figure 4.7); even when scarred, injured and distorted, the body will still create the best state of equilibrium possible, working with brilliant, innate intelligence around the damage. Figure 3.1 is an example of the adaptive nature of the body. This scar was the result of a Meckel's diverticulum operation at four months old. Always tight, raised and pulling on surrounding tissue, the scar did not cause significant problems until after

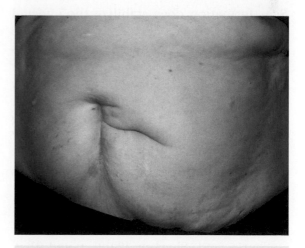

Figure 3.1
An example of the adaptive nature of the body.

three pregnancies and a gain in bodyweight. Adhesions formed under the scar and behind the umbilicus, eventually causing abdominal distortion and discomfort, and also affecting posture. As confirmed by a CT scan, during the two years prior to this photograph, adhesion formation had occurred, possibly because of keyhole surgeries (cholecystectomy and ovariectomy). No other complications were found, and a decision was made not to operate due to the risk of more adhesions forming. ScarWork was given resulting in some improvement but the adhesions were strong and deep; a medical referral to investigate the possibility of reconsidering surgery has since been requested.

How scars affect our tension/compression system

Scar formation does stabilize the affected area, but it may be chaotic: "Scar tissue formation is not selective. Scar tissue forms at the site of tissue damage, and the repair process encompasses and incorporates any type of injured tissue into the same scar. This applies to all types of tissue, including the dermis, muscles, tendons, and bone" (Guimberteau and Armstrong 2015). Functionality will, therefore, be affected by this process.

Fourie and Sharkey (2018) noted that: "Living a life results in short- and long-term adaptations due to overuse (lack of recovery), disuse (lack of activity), misuse (inappropriate activity) and traumatic events (overload).

It is when a person runs out of adaptive capacity that they often experience pain and changes in sensations in the fascial system particularly related to issues with force transmission, restrictive adhesions or scars, fibrosis and painful rigid collagenous tissues." Thus, adhesions can affect different people in different ways.

Someone who may eventually run out of adaptive capacity could be a young mother with a C-section scar. If she develops a habit of holding the baby on one hip, this can create an area of reduced mobility and tissue degeneration caused by misuse (Figure 3.2). The fascia responds to the one-sided force directed into it, collagen will be laid down along the line of force and the body shape will adapt around this one-sided positioning. Where the extra collagen fibers have been laid down, a densification of the fascia can occur, which supports the body in this activity – holding the baby on one hip – but which then has repercussions as the body compensates around the adaptation. Add to this the probable presence of adhesions from the C-section scar, which may feed into the tissues of the less mobile hip, and we see that the body is now dealing with two insults where the reduced mobility from misuse renders the body more vulnerable to the restrictive adhesions, and the body shape will change by virtue of the adaptation required. The myofascial holding patterns will now limit the ability of the body to move well in certain planes. Years later this woman may arrive at a clinic complaining of back or knee pain, and the cause of the postural patterning will be deduced from her medical history. Scar therapy to lessen the effect of the adhesions and fascia-focused work to the densification and holding patterns will usually help to restore original body shape, assist in restoration of the circulation of blood and lymph, improve functionality and reduce discomfort.

An example is illustrated in Figure 3.2, where the original complaint was low thoracic pain and numbness in the scar. For the full case study, see Chapter 11, pp. 145–147.

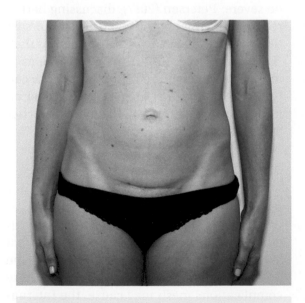

Figure 3.2
Reduced mobility from misuse renders the body more vulnerable to restrictive adhesions, and body shape will change by virtue of the adaptation required.

Working with the scarred body

It will be difficult, if not impossible, for a manual therapist to successfully realign or rebalance the body on a permanent basis when there are adhesions disrupting the normal distribution of tension, because the aberrant tensional patterns which adhesions create are often deep-seated and highly resistant to change. Therefore, it is important to work on the scar tissue first, because it is further up the chain, with the aim of softening that tissue and thus reducing the consequences further down the chain.

Even with all of a therapist's skills deployed, the process that manual therapy will start in the body – the diminishing of abnormal tension, of (strain) patterns, of structural imbalances, results that would normally cascade through the body – will be limited by adhered tissues. Rather like trying to redistribute the stuffing in a duvet that has become bunched up in the spare room after a while, normally a couple of good shakes should be effective, but if someone has repaired a tear in the duvet and caught both sides of the cover with the stitching, the filling will be unable to get past that obstruction.

Mesh and the adaptive body

A mesh is a structure introduced into the body during surgery to provide support when the body's natural support has been compromised, such as in a hernia or during pelvic floor repair. Although mesh implants can be successful, recently they have become the focus of worldwide furore, with many recipients reporting debilitating pain, in particular women treated for vaginal prolapse, with the mesh breaking through the vaginal wall and/or creating nerve damage. The acute and chronic pain resulting from this has resulted in an eruption of lawsuits. Removal of the mesh is possible but difficult; because the mesh is designed to become interwoven with the body's tissue, it literally becomes enmeshed.

It is clear that removing a mesh is far from simple but may be necessary if it is causing severe pain (Figure 3.3). However, considering the amount of tissue that has to be removed

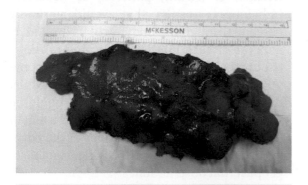

Figure 3.3

A mesh after removal. This photograph demonstrates the interweaving of the tissue into the mesh, making the latter extremely difficult to remove in cases of a painful reaction.

Photograph reproduced by kind permission of Kevin C. Petersen, M.D.

along with the mesh, there will obviously be further physical distortion and compensation around the twice-damaged area (from the insertion and removal of a foreign object), as well as further scarring, some of which will now be quite deep internally. The force distribution will be altered resulting in all the associated consequences.

There is, no doubt, much successful mesh insertion surgery. However, in those cases where the mesh is rejected, the body's inflammatory response can create adhesions. Also, when mesh moves despite the anchors applied (see below), the results can be severe; Petersen (2017), discussing hernia repairs and the contractile property of scar tissue which can lead to pain, points out that: "One of the other unfortunate side effects of mesh scar contracture is [that] the mesh can break away from its anchors and shrivel up into a wad and become ineffective as a barrier to herniation."

From the biotensegrity point of view, this practice of mesh fixation in certain operations is an issue which needs further consideration. In a detailed explanation of what a vaginal repair with mesh entails and the possible outcomes, which include those complications mesh may cause, the International Urogynecological Association (2019) advised that "Different techniques are used to implant the graft and to keep it in place. These include fixation arms that exit through a few additional small incisions at the inner thigh and/or the buttocks, or special anchors that fix the mesh to firm structures in the pelvis (such as the sacrospinous ligament)." However, our biotensegral nature lies in the context-dependent mobility of every structure in the body. As one part moves in response to internal or external forces, so the rest of the body adapts in order to maintain structural integrity and balance; it is a constantly moving and changing organism. Anchor a fixation arm of mesh to a structure and you will compromise that potential mobility. When part of the body has its freedom of movement restricted, this can and will lead to soft tissue and joint issues throughout the body, which will not necessarily appear to be connected in any way to the initial pelvic repair.

The future of mesh

Fitzgerald and Kumar (2014), in their comparison of biologic (human, bovine and porcine decellularized tissue) and synthetic mesh options, look at the properties of the different meshes on the market, and their known side effects and benefits. Different meshes affect the body in different ways and the skill is to find one with the correct strength, porosity and construction best-suited for the individual. Synthetic mesh development is moving towards the absorbable, which is "designed to be completely degraded over time." The focus of the study was the avoidance of adhesion formation and achieving a balance between minimizing it and providing an adequately strong mesh scaffold that will last long enough to generate sufficient new tissue ingrowth.

On 10 July 2018, the BBC reported that "The health watchdog NICE [National Institute for Health and Care Excellence] has already recommended that vaginal mesh operations for treating organ prolapse should largely be stopped in England" (BBC News, 2018). A review has been ordered and we await the outcome.

Box 3.1 Vaginal prolapse and problems of vaginal mesh
Niall Galloway

The vagina is shaped like a funnel, wider on the inside and narrower at the opening to allow the birthing baby an easier path. The bladder rests on the anterior vaginal wall and the rectum is supported behind the posterior wall. Vaginal walls are made of fascia, the fabric from which we are all made, a continuity of attachments that frame every tissue and organ; but the vagina is made only of fascia and, like the mouth, the vagina is lined with a moist epithelium.

Fascia is a mixture of fibers suspended in a ground substance. The fibers are dynamic, mixed with myofibroblast cells, and the ground substance is variable, able to change in response to hormonal signaling, and to local conditions, including the forces of push and pull. Like smooth bedsheets tucked in on a newly made bed, the vaginal walls are attached securely to the pelvic sidewalls, but birthing a baby can disturb the lateral attachments. The initial disturbance may be small, but once disturbed, the vagina is free to bulge to the outside (like a pocket that can be turned inside out). If surgical repair is required, the task is to reattach the vagina to the pelvic sidewall and thus restore the normal pelvic support anatomy.

continued

Once popular, vaginal mesh surgeries (as in Figure 3.4) have fallen from favor as we have learned more about vaginal fascia, wound healing and the patterns of severe mesh complications.

Surgery results in wounds that trigger myofibroblasts to their primal response: to lay down strings of collagen, fill and fix the tissues, then wind in the fibers like mini-winches to close the defect and heal the wound. If a mesh is in the wound, the fibers will become tethered to the mesh and the mini-winches will pull and deform the mesh, leading to thickening, shortening, folding and distortion of the mesh.

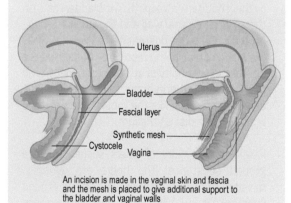

An incision is made in the vaginal skin and fascia and the mesh is placed to give additional support to the bladder and vaginal walls

Figure 3.4
Prolapse repair: anterior compartment (cystocele repair), using synthetic mesh.

A dynamic organ, the vagina is by necessity soft, accommodating and compliant for both sexual activity and childbirth. By contrast, vaginal meshes are made of plastic and, like brittle plastic bottles in the environment, resist degradation and persist for year after year. Mesh is not inert, it is unpredictable; it can react in the body

and may thicken and buckle causing increased tension and pain, and can also be a source of chronic inflammation.

Like the healthy mouth, the vagina is colonized with numerous bacteria and other organisms, thus is able to be clean, but never sterile. Mesh is prone to infections, and when they occur, it is notoriously resistant to host defences and antibiotics, and likely to persist until all of the infected mesh is surgically removed. Infection has been linked with serious mesh complications, including chronic discharge, wound separation, exposure, erosion, bleeding, shrinkage and chronic pelvic pain. Vaginal mesh, when surgically removed, does not look or feel anything like it does in the package, and its many problems make mesh products unsuitable for use, especially in sexually active women.

When a scar is the lesser of two evils

Scars need not always be perceived as damaging. For example, Kiernan (2018) states that internal derangement of the temporomandibular joint (TMJ) occurs when the articular disc is displaced from the condylar head, resulting in varying presentations and symptoms. Where TMJ disc displacement occurs without reduction (i.e. without returning to its correct position on the condyle on mouth opening), resulting in limited opening, the retrodiscal tissue, which is highly vascularized and innervated, becomes compressed between the condyle and the articular fossa. The inflammatory response to this trauma may lead to scarring of the retrodiscal tissue (Box 3.2). The blood vessels and nerves are replaced by more fibrous tissue, which forms what is known as a functioning "pseudo disc"; there is evidence that suggests the clinical situation is slightly improved for those with rather than without this adaptation (Bristela et al. 2017).

Box 3.2 Intraoral and dental scars and their effect on the body
Tracey Kiernan

Few papers have been published regarding intraoral wounds and the classification of wound healing in the mouth. We do know that the healing of oral mucosa differs from skin healing in that it is usually faster and generates less scar tissue (Okazi et al. 2002). Healing with reduced or no scar formation is often believed to be due to the intraoral environment. However, research has shown a similarity between intraoral and fetal wound healing. These both differ from general postnatal healing because of variations within the extracellular matrix, cellular mediators and inflammatory response (Larson et al. 2010). We can learn from these different processes and apply that knowledge to scars on the body.

The effect of dental scars on the TMJ and the rest of the body

There are many different types of tissue in the mouth that heal in different ways. For example, wounds to the palate usually heal with minimal scars whereas an incision in the buccal mucosa will more often result in scar formation (Larjava et al. 2011).

Intraoral scar tissue formation may range from minimal or no scar tissue to severe fibrosis that can result in a trismus. Adhesions within the muscles of mastication may contribute to trigeminal neuralgia through compression of the trigeminal nerve.

Scars, adhesions or restrictions in the muscles of mastication (masseter, temporalis, lateral and medial pterygoids) can affect the delicate balance of the TMJ (Figure 3.5) and thereby impact further down the myofascial chain. The TMJ

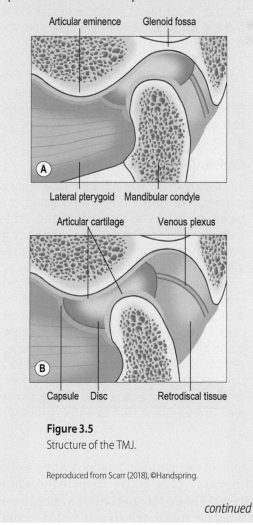

Figure 3.5
Structure of the TMJ.

Reproduced from Scarr (2018), ©Handspring.

continued

shares an interconnected relationship to the transverse fascial planes, including the hyoid, respiratory diaphragm and pelvic floor, as well as the shoulder girdle and pelvis.

Many of those structures are connected through the "deep front line", a myofascial continuity proposed by Tom Myers (2011) that shows the fascial connections from the cranium, through the muscles of mastication, the tissues of the thoracic cavity to the iliopsoas, adductors and deep toe flexors of the feet.

From these new models we may begin to consider the global impact of dental scars on everything from the TMJ to the balance of the pelvis to the stability of the knees and ankles and the arches of the feet.

Conclusion

The healing of wounds in the intraoral cavity is a subject that invites further investigation. In a recent article on TMJ tensegrity (2018), James Earls, the author of *Born to Walk*, wrote: "Putting everything into context for our clients is not easy. We must assess skeletal relationships, interpret soft tissue patterns and be mindful of emotional contexts. We should not be surprised when we work on the low back and the jaw eases, or vice versa – they are linked! When a client is complaining of foot issues and their pronation or supination is affected, why not check the jaw for a holding pattern. If we cannot balance the quadratus lumborum to ease a tilted ribcage, can we start to relax the area by first exploring the jaw?"

One of the contraindications when working with scars is to be aware of where the scarred/adhered tissue has become an incontrovertible part of the body's structure. For example,

without it a joint might be less stable. On one occasion, when I was working with Healing Hands Network[2], a client took off his shoes and socks, then peeled off an extra layer of padding from his rather small right foot. On closer inspection, the plantar aspect was a mass of scars, and the great and first toes had been removed by the same grenade which had caused the plantar damage (Figure 3.6). The other toes had moved medially to compensate, and in doing so had created a compact unit that took the strain of walking reasonably well. This was a brilliant example of the body adapting to unusual circumstances. If I had tried to free up the scars, I would have affected the balance of the adapted foot and possibly the integrity of the structure. He would not have thanked me.

The human body will always adapt to its injuries, and the formation of scars and adhesions is an almost inevitable consequence of this process. Homeostasis and the drive towards a more balanced state is built into our very being. However, such tissues are often associated with unwanted signs and symptoms, including pain, and therapeutic approaches which successfully address these issues are an essential part of everyday practice. When a scar is contraindicated for work, the body's own adaptations will be the optimum in the circumstances, although there may be interventions that can assist in pain reduction.

---

2   http://www.healinghandsnetwork.org.uk. This charity is dedicated to the relief of suffering from the mental, physical and emotional aftereffects of war, treating people overseas and in UK forces.

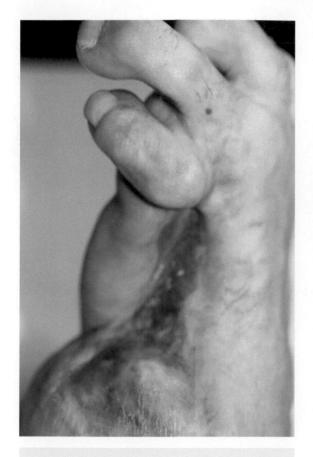

Figure 3.6
The body can adapt to the most difficult of circumstances.

References

BBC News (2018). *Immediate stop to NHS mesh operations*. Available at: https://www.bbc.co.uk/news/health-44763673[accessed 6 December 2018].

Bristela, M., Schmid-Schwap, M., Eder, J., Reichenberg, G., Kundi, M., Piehslinger, E., and Robinson, S. (2017). Magnetic resonance imaging of temporomandibular joint with anterior disk dislocation without reposition – long-term results. *Clinical Oral Investigations*. 21:237–245.

Earls, J. (2018). TMJ Tensegrity Module: TMJ Therapy®. TMJ2 Blend Therapy Training (appendix 1) [unpublished].

Fitzgerald, J. F., and Kumar, A. S. (2014). *Biologic versus Synthetic Mesh Reinforcement: What are the Pros and Cons?* Clinics in Colon and Rectal Surgery. Available at: https://www.ncbi.nlm.nih.gov/pmc/articles/PMC4477030/[accessed 10 December 2018].

Fourie, W., and Sharkey, J. (2018). *S.C.A.R. Therapy Workshop Manual* (page 8). Edinburgh Training and Conference Venue, Edinburgh, UK. 25–26 June 2018.

Galloway, N. (2018). Personal correspondence.

Guimberteau, J. C., and Armstrong, C. (2015). *Architecture of Human Living Fascia*. Edinburgh, UK: Handspring Publishing.

International Urogynecological Association (2019). *Vaginal repair with mesh. Your Pelvic Floor*. Available at: https://www.yourpelvicfloor.org/conditions/vaginal-repair-with-mesh [accessed 2 January 2019].

Kiernan, T. (2018). Personal correspondence.

Larjava, H., Wiebe, C., Gallant-Behm, C., Hart, D. A., Heino, J., and Häkkinen, L. (2011). Exploring scarless healing of oral soft tissues. *Journal of the Canadian Dental Association*. 77:b18.

Larson, B. J., Longaker, M. T., and Lorenz, H. P. (2010). Scarless fetal wound healing: a basic science review. *Plastic and Reconstructive Surg*ery. 126:1172–1180.

Myers, T. W. (2011). *Anatomy Trains*. London, UK: Urban & Fischer.

Okazi, M., Yoshimura, K., Uchida, G., and Harii, K. (2002). Elevated expression of hepatocyte and keratinocyte growth factor in cultured buccal mucosa derived fibro-blasts compared with normal skin derived fibroblasts. *Foetal Dermatological Science*. 30:108–115.

Peterson, K. C. (2017). *An Informal Hernia Mesh Literature Review*. Available at: https://www.noinsurancesurgery.com/hernia/hernia-mesh-literature-review.htm [accessed 1 December 2018].

Scarr, G. (2018). *Biotensegrity. The Structural Basis of Life* (2nd edition). Edinburgh, UK: Handspring Publishing.

Chapter 4

Modeling the effects of scars and adhesions on the body

Graham Scarr

Introduction

Biotensegrity is refreshing because it enables us to examine the organization, mechanics and consequences of scars and adhesions from a viewpoint that is based on first principles. This chapter explains how the basic rules of physics guide the self-assembly, organization and motion of complex anatomy, using simple models to demonstrate how changes in one part of a system can have a profound effect on other parts some distance away.

Biotensegrity is a different approach to understanding the body, and this chapter starts by examining the effects of these basic principles on the organization and motion of complex living tissues. We will also look at the significance of structural heterarchies, force-transfer and closed-chain kinematics, and show how they change conventional ideas about what scars and adhesions really are. A different appreciation of the terms "health" and "dysfunction" offers a more objective approach to understanding the problems of our patients and how to treat them.

The organization of structure

The human body is a mechanical unit, and a very effective one at that. It can move with the minimum of effort and operate for up to a 100 years or more, and does so with little external help. As a growing embryo, it regulates its own development and emerges as a fully formed organism, but there is no blueprint or programmed design. Although the genetic code has been assumed to fulfill this role, it is simply a source of information in the manufacture of proteins and does not directly determine how or why such complicated molecules behave in the ways in which they do. Development is a naturally evolving process that results from the actions of physical forces between molecules and the tissues that they form; these forces come in two types – those that attract and those that repel.

At the most basic level, there are many ways in which atoms can interact with each other, but they can all be categorized into those that attract or those that repel. These forces always coexist, causing atoms to assemble into structures that we recognize as rigid crystals and more flexible molecules (e.g. amino acids), and they do so because of some fundamental principles of self-organization. These include: 1) geodesic geometry, where these forces always take the shortest path, traveling in straight lines; 2) close-packing, where the atoms arrange themselves into the most stable configurations possible; and 3) minimal energy, where everything happens in the simplest and most efficient way (Levin 2006, Scarr 2018B).

The same principles also govern how simple molecules interact with each other and form more complex arrangements, and also apply to the self-assembly of all natural structures at every scale, no matter how complicated. Such invisible molecules can then arrange themselves into tangible anatomical structures that transmit their own higher level forces of tension and compression as part of their functionality, for example, collagen fibers, proteoglycans, fascia and bones. The existence of each structural entity is thus dependent on the totality of forces that flow within it, and which in turn manifest themselves through its particular architecture. Even though the system becomes enormously complicated, each of its anatomical parts is formed according to the same principles and relies on the integrated balance of forces to maintain its stability. Tension and compression are then separated into distinct structural pathways at multiple levels that ultimately define the human body as a tensegrity structure (Levin 2006, Ingber et al. 2014).

The omnidirectional heterarchy

Biotensegrity implicitly recognizes the value of these fundamental principles as a better way of understanding structural anatomy, helping us appreciate the energy-efficient heterarchical organization that emerges from their interactions. Every molecule, cell, fiber, tissue, bone, muscle, organ or joint becomes a modular close-packed unit that is nested within and linked to all those surrounding it at every size-scale (Esteve-Altava 2017) (Figure 4.1). In other words, living tissues are intrinsically heterarchical, and each anatomical part consists of smaller parts, which themselves contain even smaller parts,

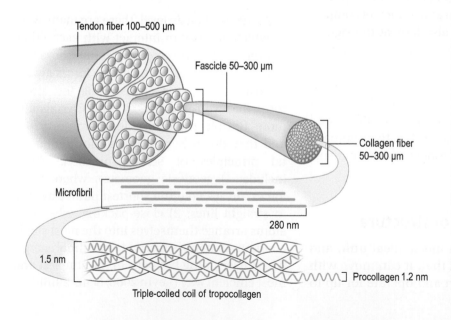

Tendon fiber 100–500 μm

Fascicle 50–300 μm

Collagen fiber 50–300 μm

Microfibril

280 nm

1.5 nm

Procollagen 1.2 nm

Triple-coiled coil of tropocollagen

Figure 4.1

A simplified heterarchy consisting of procollagen, tropocollagen, fibril, fiber, fascicle and tendon.

Modified from Scarr (2010) © Elsevier.

and all of these parts are integrated into a complete structural and functional unit. They reduce mass, increase strength and optimize the load-bearing ability, and provide a mechanism for dissipating potentially damaging stresses down through the multilevel system, thus rendering them harmless (Simon 1962). This omnidirectional continuity also enables each part to influence other parts some distance away and explains why the formation of scars and adhesions can have such widespread consequences.

Heterarchical principles are neatly demonstrated through the construction of simple tensegrities, and the model in Figure 4.2A shows that the end of each strut (the node) has four cables attached to it (creating pin-joints), where the tensional forces become concentrated. Figure 4.2B is a simple heterarchical model of the end of one of these struts, with both the strut and its four cables modeled as a chain of similar tensegrity modules each

connected together in a similar way. It can be observed that the number of links between the strut and its cables has increased, enabling the tensional stresses between them to be distributed over a much larger field, making the total structure much stronger, thus enabling it to function within a greater range of operating conditions. Most importantly, every part has a direct influence on all the other parts.

Anatomical textbooks, however, have in general conformed to a hierarchical system of large important structures followed by smaller and less significant ones, and have failed to emphasize their integrated relationships. We have, for example, a lot of information concerning bones and muscles, but less regarding how the fascial tissues and forces within them contribute to their functions. A heterarchical perspective recognizes that every small part makes an important contribution to the whole, and that the forces of tension and compression can be transferred

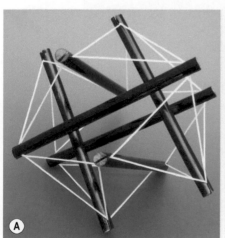

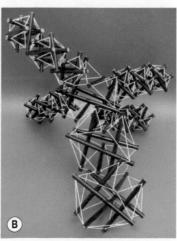

Figure 4.2

(A) T-icosa model showing the four tension cables attached to the end (node) of each strut; (B) a two-level heterarchical model of a single node showing the increased number of links between the cables and strut, and how the forces are distributed throughout.

throughout the body in a definable way (Turvey and Fonseca 2014).

Considering structural biology from an integrated, whole-body perspective thus provides a conceptual platform from where to examine its functions and pathologies, and inevitably means studying those mechanisms which cause them. Living tissues are constantly changing their shapes and positions, and tensegrity nicely models this behavior because the mechanics that underlie movements are exactly the same.

The geometry of motion

Closed kinematic chains (CKCs) have long been used in mechanical engineering because they provide a simple and efficient mechanism with multiple applications. They are also ubiquitous in biology, constituting the basic mechanics of the tensegrity model, and are crucial to understanding the behavior of scars and adhesions. CKCs couple multiple parts ('bars') into continuous mechanical loops with each one influencing the position of all the others in the system, enabling the controlled transfer and amplification (or attenuation) of force, speed and kinetic energy (Levin et al. 2017) (Figure 4.3).

Kinematics concerns the geometry of motion, and the simplest geometric arrangement that enables the structure to control this is the planar four-bar, where the length

and position of each linkage bar determines the position and movement of all the others. The angular relationships between them define its mechanical properties and enable useful comparisons between different parts of the body, and other species to be made

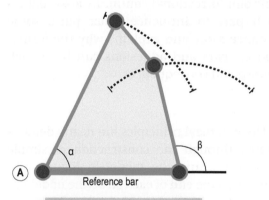

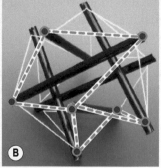

Figure 4.3

(A) A four-bar shape showing the pin-joints, trajectories and limits of three moving bars in relation to a fixed reference bar, and how the motion of each bar is controlled by the relative positions of all the others, with the changing relationship between the angles (α and β) defining its mechanical properties. (B) A T-icosa showing some of the stable three-bar (white) and flexible four-bar (blue dotted) closed kinematic chains that regulate changes in shape.

(Muller 1996). By comparison, three-bar triangular arrangements can be relatively rigid and are important because of their stability, while those with five or more bars are unstable on their own but are crucial to more complicated systems. The constructivist artist, Theo Jansen, neatly illustrates the functional benefits of coupling multiple three- and four-bar CKCs by using his autonomous "Strandbeest" creatures that walk along beaches in the Netherlands, powered entirely by the wind (Figure 4.4).

In a biological context, the functional value of CKCs to normal physiology has been recognized since at least the 18th century, and is well described in the feeding mechanisms of fish, birds and crustaceans, but has only recently attracted significant attention in humans (Levin et al. 2017, Scarr and Harrison 2017). For example: the cruciate ligaments within the knee form part of a crossed four-bar mechanism that efficiently guides the motion of the femur and tibia in relation to each other (Figure 4.5A); the configuration of connective tissues within the fingers that process information (force and direction) perform their own logical computations and switch the system between different functional states, thereby changing the position of the bones in relation to each other (Valero-Cuevas et al. 2007) (Figure 4.5B); and the multiarticular limb muscles that couple multiple joints together, enable forces and power to be transferred

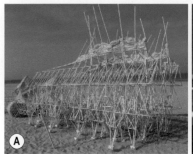
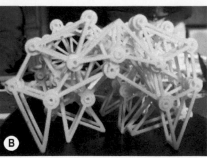
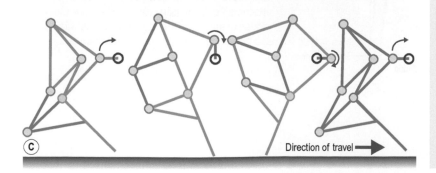

Figure 4.4

(A) Theo Janssen's Strandbeest creature (reproduced courtesy of ©Theo Jansen). (B) A similar model showing the interlinked closed kinematic chains (CKCs) (courtesy Theo Jansen). (C) The basic three- and four-bar CKCs that control changes in limb shape and movement (reproduced from Scarr (2018B) ©Handspring).

Direction of travel ➡

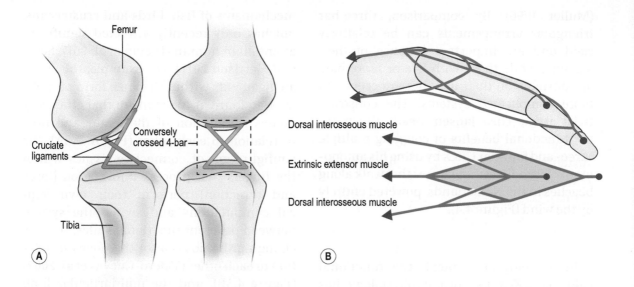

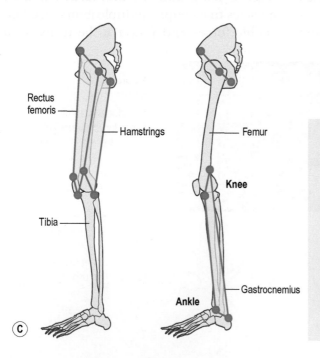

Figure 4.5

Simple four-bar systems: (A) the cruciate ligaments form a crossed four-bar arrangement in the knee; (B) the extensor tendon network in the middle finger indicating the direction of muscle tension (arrows), Winslow's rhombus (pink four-bar) and multibar connective tissues (red dots indicate key bone attachments); (C) multiarticular muscles guide the motion of the hip, knee and ankle and enable forces and power to be transferred between them.

Redrawn from Levin et al. (2017); not to scale.

from one part of the body to another in a controlled way (Van Ingen Schenau 1994) (Figure 4.5C).

Such interconnected, omnidirectional CKC systems are intrinsic to the regulation of motion and enable the tissues to respond instantly to unexpected or rapidly changing conditions, and in ways which would otherwise be impossible, with the nervous system acting in synergy and at a higher level of control (Wilson and Kiely 2016).

At first glance, however, such arrangements may appear to be little more than complex lever systems, but this description does not do them justice in a biological context because of their heterarchical nature. Here, each modular bar is made from numerous smaller modules, and the term "pin-joint" refers to the multiscale tensegrity connections between one structural entity and another (Figure 4.2). The bars then relate to passive structures such as collagen fibers, bones, tendons, ligaments, fascia, scars and adhesions, or active tension generators such as muscles, and together they form an integrated motion system that extends throughout the body (Figure 4.6). Each one influences all those that it is connected to in a continuous, moment-by-moment transition that transfers forces between the simplest and most complex parts, and with multiple mechanical properties that become collectively optimized throughout the entire system (Levin 2006).

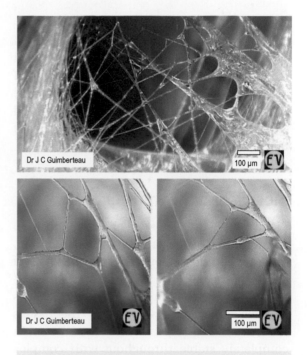

Figure 4.6

The irregular fractal-like CKC organization ('microvacuoles') of the extracellular matrix in vivo as revealed within the (expanded) fascia of the upper limb; the two bottom pictures show how changes in matrix tension cause the individual fiber bundles ('bars') to coalesce and separate, thus changing the geometry (shape) of the entire CKC system.

Reproduced from Guimberteau and Armstrong (2015) ©Handspring.

Such a heterarchical organization reveals that there are no fixed fulcrums, bending moments or shear stresses, and that the concept of levers has no place in a biological context. Most importantly, each structural entity (bar) is either under tension or compression and has its own unique properties that determine how the higher level structure behaves. It is thus the efficient local separation and higher level integration of these forces within the global architecture that ultimately define these coupled closed chain systems as the underlying mechanics of tensegrity, living structures and movement.

Motion and the transfer of forces

Movement is the result of a change in position or orientation of one part in relation to another, and must be carried out in a controlled way if it is to be purposeful, with the closed chain/ tensegrity architecture indicating how this can be achieved. It shows how the tissues themselves can regulate motion and remain completely stable throughout with complex control tasks outsourced directly into the structure and efficiently reducing the amount of effort required by the nervous system (Turvey and Fonseca 2014) (Figure 4.5). The tension and compressional forces that enable this to happen are then transferred (flow) along specific anatomical pathways (bars) as part of normal functioning, but any change in this configuration will alter their distribution and therefore has the potential to cause problems.

The distribution of forces

Living tissues are dynamic structures where everything is changing and adapting to those changes over time. Bones are being continuously remodeled by the cells within them and in response to forces imposed from their environment (Wolff's Law). Muscles waste away if

they are not being used or they become stronger when exercised; the extracellular matrix and connective tissues reorganize themselves according to the prevailing stresses (Davis's Law); and molecules are continually interacting with one other and undergoing transformation in complex ways. The stability and behavior of each one is thus totally dependent on the changing balance of the forces acting both upon and within it.

Muscles provide the power required for movement but the distribution of their tensional force is over a much greater anatomical field than is usually appreciated. Tendons, ligaments and inter/extra-muscular fascial tissues are all involved in the transmission of tension to bones, other muscles, aponeuroses and the deep fascia (Schleip et al. 2012), and which are themselves continuous with the fibrous extracellular matrix that links them all together. Because there is no real distinction between where one part ends and the other begins (at the micro-level), physical forces are able to flow easily within this basic level of tissue organization (Guimberteau and Armstrong 2016) (Figure 4.6). So although we may be more familiar with the arrangements of bones, muscles, tendons and ligaments provided in textbooks, the omnidirectional heterarchy of force pathways that link these elements together is far more complex and unique to each individual, and the cells that create it are an integral part of this.

Most cells are involved in the cyclic processes of growing, differentiating, reproducing and dying, thus changing the structure and mechanical behavior of their associated tissues over time. The tensegrity cytoskeletons within fibroblasts and muscle cells, for example, are constantly generating tension and transferring it to the surrounding extracellular matrix as part of normal function (Ingber et al. 2014); and because muscles are always active, even when at rest, they are better considered as dynamic regulators of connective tissue tension than mere motors of movement (Masi and Hannon 2009). Such intrinsic tissue tension (prestress) is hugely important because it removes any slack from the tissues, primes the system for action and enables it to respond instantly to changing forces from anywhere in the CKC network. It is also a defining characteristic of tensegrity, and the physiological consequences of such force transfer are implicit to our understanding of and the treatment of scars and adhesions (Levin 2006).

The patterns of motion

Movement is the means that we use to express life – whether walking, talking, working or playing – and the appearance of a regular pattern of motion is characteristic of an efficient regulatory system (Iosa et al. 2013). Recognizable patterns pervade the entire field of biology, and every practitioner is doubtless aware how they can change between normal and abnormal. For example, a person carrying a heavy bag on one shoulder will automatically adjust their posture and change the usual patterns of motion of the head, neck, shoulders and pelvis during walking. The uneven weight distribution alters the balance of forces and causes the body-wide CKC/tensegrity geometry to adjust itself to the changing situation, leading to compensatory changes in neural/muscle activity. When one part changes, everything changes, which is a normal functional adaptation to changing circumstances.

These scenarios of shifting posture occur thousands of times each day when walking, manipulating an object or even chewing on one side of the jaw, but can become a problem if a particular pattern predominates. Certain tissues may be loaded in ways that they are unable to sustain, with the resulting micro-trauma initiating a cellular response that potentially leads to inflammation, fibrosis and increased tissue stiffness. A change in the normal distribution of forces within one region can then set up a mechanical conflict with an adjacent or distant region (through the CKC network), producing signs and symptoms which may otherwise appear unfathomable; the same can also happen with tissues that have been traumatized (Tabibian et al. 2017).

Scars are typically a result of injuries that cut or penetrate the skin (including surgery), with the inflammatory and self-healing processes that naturally follow leading to changes in the local tissue organization (Kollmmansberger et al. 2018). Consequently, the mechanical properties and response of those tissues to the forces that flow through them during movement will be altered, and may adversely influence the behavior of other tissues which are

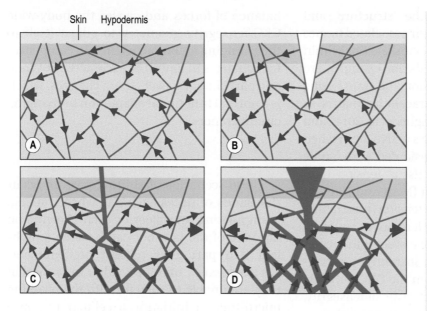

Skin Hypodermis

Figure 4.7
Proposed stages in the development of a scar and adhesion following surgery. The small red arrows indicate the flow of forces through the subcutaneous fascial tissues (purple) when tensioned in a particular direction (large red arrows): (A) a normal pattern of fibers within the extracellular matrix and fascial network; (B) surgery changes the pattern of forces as they continue to follow the path of least resistance; (C) body movements cause the resultant tensional forces to move deeper as the tissues become more fibrotic; (D) the developing adhesion reinforces itself in a positive feedback loop that changes the tissue mechanics.

some distance away. Adhesions can develop between tissues that previously transferred tensional forces along specific pathways, but which have now become disrupted and have altered the normal pattern of force distribution (Figure 4.7). As they continue to develop in response to the forces that flow through them (Davis's Law), they become reinforced through a positive feedback loop that spreads their influence even deeper into the tissues. So although we often consider scars and adhesions to be pathological because of the problems they cause, they are simply reflecting changes in the CKC/tensegrity/tissue architecture and distributing a different pattern of forces.

Health and dysfunction: What is the difference?

At this point, we should take a step back from our instinctive response to disease (at least for a moment) and reconsider what is meant by such terms as dysfunction, injury and pathology. These words can be misleading from a biotensegrity perspective because they evoke images of harm, damage and abnormality, and imply that something must be wrong and that it needs fixing. Certainly, from the patient's or client's point of view, they are in pain or something is not working quite right and the practitioner needs to have empathy and compassion for their situation, but a treatment approach which simply fixes problems is omitting something important and may not provide the best care for that individual.

Mechanical forces (tension and compression) do not flow in a haphazard manner but always follow the path of least resistance, and their efficient distribution through omnidirectional heterarchy is ultimately what regulates normal patterns of motion (Figures 4.3–4.6). Indeed, one of the characteristics of life is the ability of the body to transform its architecture in ways that enable mechanical forces to flow more easily, and such a constantly evolving system applies to every aspect of a developing and self-sustaining organism (Bejan 2016).

Living tissues can thus be considered to function in exactly the same way in a healthy body as in a dysfunctioning body, in the sense that the physiological processes that maintain them are always governed by the same basic principles, always moving towards a lower energy state, just as water flows downhill (Levin 2006). Even though homeostasis is built into the system, a change in the distribution of forces through and around a scar or adhesion will inevitably shift the tissues away from their normal operating parameters and may lead to problems; but as they are simply acting within a different set of spatial constraints and displaying a different pattern of behavior, we are the ones who make the value judgments about health and dysfunction, and not the biology (Scarr 2018A, 2018B).

Treatment of whatever sort is about more than just releasing tissue tension, improving mobility or fixing problems – it is a dynamic interactive process that changes the tissue geometry, that is, changes the CKC/tensegrity architecture. The body's self-organizing processing systems respond to this in the most energy-efficient (and only) manner they can and move towards a different state of health; an understanding of biotensegrity provides the rationale for this.

Conclusion

The architecture of flow

Biotensegrity changes the way that we look at life and its problems, with scars and adhesions demonstrating the consequences of self-healing efforts that have 'run away' with themselves; but there is nothing inherently malicious about them. They are simply physical representations of the forces that flow through them, and they develop in response to inflammatory conditions and changes in the patterns of tension and compression within the local environment. Such forces always follow the path of least resistance, with the resulting architecture forming in response to driving, motion-induced currents and local constraints in the environment through which they flow. That a structural change in one part of the body can lead to problems in another is unfortunate, but from a biotensegrity perspective is just a local conflict of interest within a complex system that is constantly evolving and trying to maintain its dynamic stability.

Chapter 4

References

Bejan, A. (2016). Life and evolution as physics. *Communicative and Integrative Biology*. 9:e1172159.

Esteve-Altava, B. (2017). In search of morphological modules: a systematic review. *Biological Reviews*. 92:1332–1347.

Guimberteau, J. C., and Armstrong, C. (2015). *Architecture of human living fascia: the extracellular matrix and cells revealed through endoscopy*. Edinburgh, UK: Handspring.

Ingber, D. E., Wang, N., and Stamenović, D. (2014). Tensegrity, cellular biophysics and the mechanics of living systems. *Reports on Progress in Physics*. 77:046603.

Iosa, M., Fusco, A., Marchetti, F., Morone, G., Caltagirone, C., Paolucci, S., and Peppe, A. (2013). The golden ratio of gait harmony: repetitive proportions of repetitive gait phases. *BioMed Research International*. 2013:918642.

Kollmannsberger, P., Bidan, C. M., Dunlop, J. W. C., Fratzl, P., and Vogel, V. (2018). Tensile forces drive a reversible fibroblast-to-myofibroblast transition during tissue growth in engineered clefts. *Science Advances*. 4:eaao4881.

Levin, S. M. (2006). Tensegrity: the new biomechanics. In: Hutson, M., and Ellis, R. (eds), *Textbook of musculoskeletal medicine*. Oxford, UK: Oxford University Press.

Levin, S. M., Lowell de Solórzano, S., and Scarr, G. (2017). The significance of closed kinematic chains to biological movement and dynamic stability. *Journal of Bodywork and Movement Therapies*. 21:664–672.

Masi, A. T., and Hannon, J. C. (2009). Human resting muscle tone (HRMT): narrative introduction and modern concepts. *Journal of Bodywork and Movement Therapies*. 12:320–332.

Muller, M. (1996). A novel classification of planar four-bar linkages and its application to the mechanical analysis of animal systems. *Philosophical Transactions of the Royal Society of London B*. 351:689–720.

Scarr, G. (2010). Simple geometry in complex organisms. *Journal of Bodywork and Movement Therapies*. 14(4):424–444.

Scarr, G. (2018A). Health and disease: what is the difference? In: Pilat, A. (ed.), *Fascia: Scientific Advances*. Proceedings of the 28th Jornadas de Fisioterapia Conference, 1–3 March 2018, pp. 219–225. Madrid, Spain: Escuela Universitaria de Fisioterapia de la Once.

Scarr, G. (2018B). *Biotensegrity. The Structural Basis of Life* (2nd edition). Edinburgh, UK: Handspring Publishing.

Scarr, G., and Harrison, H. (2017). Examining the temporo-mandibular joint from a biotensegrity perspective: a change in thinking. *Journal of Applied Biomedicine*. 15:55–62.

Schleip, R., Findley, T. W., Chaitow, L., and Huijing P. A. (eds) (2012). *Fascia: the tensional network of the human body*. Edinburgh, UK: Elsevier.

Simon, H. A. (1962). The architecture of complexity. *Proceedings of the American Philosophical Society*. 106:467–482.

Tabibian, N., Swehli, E., Boyd, A., Umbreen, A., and Tabibian, J. H. (2017). Abdominal adhesions: a practical review of an often overlooked entity. *Annals of Medicine and Surgery*. 15:9–13.

Turvey, M. T., and Fonseca, S. T. (2014). The medium of haptic perception: a tensegrity hypothesis. *Journal of Motor Behavior*. 46:143–187.

Valero-Cuevas, F. J., Yi, J. W., Brown, D., McNamara III, R. V., Paul, C., and Lipson, H. (2007). The tendon network of the fingers performs anatomical computation at a macroscopic scale. *Transactions on Biomedical Engineering*. 54:1161–1166.

Van Ingen Schenau, G. J. (1994). Proposed actions of bi-articular muscles and the design of hindlimbs of bi- and quadrupeds. *Human Movement Science*. 13:665–681.

Wilson, J., and Kiely, J. (2016). The multifunctional foot in athletic movement: extraordinary feats by our extraordinary feet. *Human Movement*. 17:15–20.

Chapter 5

The unreasonable effectiveness of light touch

Leonid Blyum

Part 1: Where we are now

Introduction

"The Unreasonable Effectiveness of Mathematics" is one of the most famous articles in the history of physics and math. In 1960, Nobel laureate Eugene Wigner expressed his fascination for how the tools of mathematics had served the natural sciences and engineering so well for several centuries, with no apparent reason for being so effective. He pointed out that humanity has been extremely fortunate to benefit from mathematical tools, despite not understanding why they work so well (Wigner 1960).

We are in a similar situation in the field of bodywork and manual therapies. For centuries, light-touch applications have been working amazingly well for different methods and therapies. Worldwide, numerous practitioners employ subtle manual interventions, thus helping millions of people with ailments. However, we have yet to fully appreciate the reasons behind the effectiveness of light touch and therefore account for its value and significance.

Where do we belong?

The first step is to ask ourselves, "How reasonable is light-touch effectiveness?" and to distinguish between reasonable, proportional, linear and plausible statements versus those appearing as unreasonable, disproportionate, non-linear and implausible. We know through personal experience that light touch works. We observe people with ailments voting for bodywork practitioners with their feet and wallets. We can feel light touch at work – under our own hands. However, we have to acknowledge that we still remain puzzled about the reasons behind its effectiveness. This lack of understanding carries an additional price: it isolates and consigns light-touch therapies to a place outside the official domain of medicine.

By making claims for the structural transformation of established scar tissue through light touch, we are making bold and scientifically unreasonable statements which defy the conventional linear scale of proportionality between cause and effect. We cannot pretend that these are weak and ordinary statements. The opposition is clear: from the scientific perspective of the 21st century, light-touch therapy applied to scars should never work.

The reasons are self-evident. What is a scar? It is a tightly packed band of collagen that has an extremely high tensile force of several Newtons per square millimeter. The light touch of a manual practitioner is approximately one hundred times less than the tensile force required to induce any breaks within those tight collagen bundles. Naturally, for skeptics, any positive declarations concerning light-touch scar therapy make no scientific sense whatsoever.

Observing the language

A light-touch therapist who claims to release/mold/soften a scar sounds very unreasonable from a scientifically rational point of view, as if making a 100-fold super effectiveness claim. Are we facing this challenge or hiding from it?

To date, bodyworkers hide from this dilemma by providing linear explanations (stretch/melt/mobilize/release) to their highly non-linear 100-fold super-effectiveness claims, where light-touch techniques transform tissues which are 100-fold stronger than the pressure applied. This linear language confusion is perfectly understandable. As bodyworkers, we trust our kinesthetic sense, internal vision, feel, touch and physical connection, but simultaneously tend to be rather loose with our language. Working within the scientific realm implies precision, of understanding the context of the terminology we deploy to conveying meaning.

Are we, as light-touch therapists, unreasonable in a good or a bad sense? If we are being unreasonable in a bad sense then we have become lost in our own storytelling and are ignoring the reality of proportional, linear responses, where light touch cannot

have an impact that amounts to one hundred times its original pressure. However, if we are being unreasonable in a good sense then we have found the secret algorithm for the disproportionate, non-linear effects that are 100-fold greater than those stipulated by linear expectations. It is only when we realize the extraordinary scale of our claims that we can move to the next step.

Proving the non-linear effectiveness of light touch

Claims concerning a 100-fold non-linear effect imply that we are dealing with a class of soft phenomena, that is, we cannot expect significant effects every single time. We must be humble and begin building our case for light touch carefully and systematically by showing that non-linear effects of 100-fold magnitude occur frequently enough to be taken seriously, meriting further exploration rather than being dismissed as mere flukes.

In this age of evidence-based medicine, a skeptic may demand that bodyworkers provide proof supporting their unreasonable claims. Fortunately, in linear thinking, the 100-fold scar tissue response to light-touch forces that are only one-hundredth of the necessary strength are so wildly implausible that the logical structure of the argument flips completely.

Usually, when a newly made claim is plausible and reasonable to a certain extent, proof of effectiveness is expected, requiring a percentage of successful outcomes to reach some critical threshold of statistical and clinical significance within a large number of cases. However, when the claim is wildly unreasonable then the burden of proof is altered. Thus, to activate the validity of our claim requires only a handful of the unreasonable and implausible precedents to have actually happened. This logically inverted path to proof is known as the "disproof of implausibility" (Figure 5.1).

Highly plausible claims do not require much proof (if any). Take this example from the field of rehabilitation: "It is likely that contractures...[of] the soft tissues arise from the muscle being maintained in a shortened position. It is possible, but not absolutely

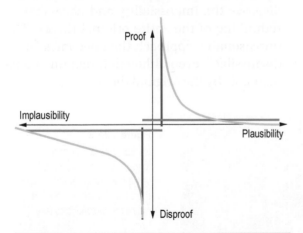

Figure 5.1

Graphic representation of the reasonable proof-plausibility relationship versus the logically inverted route towards proving the impossible.

proven, that maintaining a joint through a full range of movement may prevent the longer-term development of soft tissue contractures. The frequency of the stretch...that is required to prevent contractures is unknown" (Barnes and Johnson 2008).

Even after several hundred years of its use there is no evidence proving the positive effects of stretching on the prevention and reduction of contractures, but because this reasoning is highly plausible, stretching remains the mainstay of physical rehabilitation, despite the absence of proof.

Conversely, a low-plausibility claim that defies common sense and established scientific belief faces stern opposition and demands a much greater level of proof. These demands are impossibly high to meet in practice. This is the situation with light-touch bodywork. We have done ourselves a huge disservice by making claims of "releasing the adhesions" through minimal force. Upon these low rungs of plausibility it is impossible to meet the standards of evidence imposed via double-blind, homogeneous groups and inter-rater reliability studies. Consequently, our light-touch claims are dismissed by scientists.

Our only way to achieve recognition is by acknowledging that our claims of 100-fold super-effectiveness of light-touch pressure place us in the domain of the implausible, one which operates differently to that of the plausibility, where the more wildly implausible the claim then proportionally less is the evidence required to disprove its impossibility, thus granting us a tremendous opportunity. We don't have to labor through thousands of cases compiling percentages of high statistical probability, we need only demonstrate the disproof of implausibility via a handful of documented, observable precedents which illustrate the possibility of the impossible.

Where is the evidence?

Figure 5.2A shows a patient presenting with scarring following surgery for a necrotic colon (7 years previously) with two areas of knotting and adhesion to abdominal muscles that caused linea alba separation, restricted diaphragmatic motion and limited respiratory excursion. Following 20 hours of light-touch therapy, both knots loosened and straightened, the abdominal muscles were less constrained with reduced linea alba separation, and diaphragmatic excursion had improved (Figure 5.2B).

Do these illustrations of structural transformations of scar morphology provide sufficient proof of the validity of the light-touch approach? Absolutely. "Why?" I hear you ask. "Isn't this just anecdotal evidence? Aren't those some accidental spontaneous reactions? Don't we need stronger 'proper' statistics showing dramatic prevalence of the positive results?" Such a critique is applicable in the domain of the ordinary and linear, but remember that we are in the non-linear domain of the impossible and the unreasonable, where one-hundredth of the plausible pressure should never transform a long-standing scar. And yet it does (thus inverting the statistics).

A handful of successful precedents from the unreasonable approach are sufficient to disprove the impossibility and necessitate a rethinking of the entire original theory. The unreasonable approach then becomes "non-dismissible", even although it remains unexplainable by the original theory.

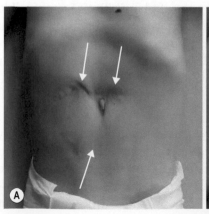 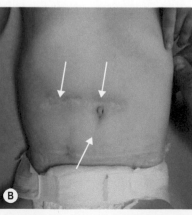

Figure 5.2A,B
(A) Abdominal scarring following surgery; (B) the same scarring after light-touch therapy. The arrows indicate major transformations (see text).

Summary: Where we are now

The light-touch impact on scars demonstrates precedents of the disproportionate 100-fold effects. The adhesions release claim is a misleading description that falsely implies the linearity of the response of fibrotic tissues, thus creating the impression of something ordinary and reasonable taking place, which is not the case with light touch. When non-linear tissues give a 100-fold response to small, one-hundredth strength impacts in what appears to be a linear manner, then that is what is extraordinary, strange and unreasonable!

In order to progress further, we bodyworkers need a deeper non-linear understanding of our kinesthetic experiences and must become non-linearity-informed. The next section explores light-touch effects from such a perspective via the formulation of the non-linear-informed light-touch bodywork hypothesis.

Part 2: Non-linear informed light-touch bodywork hypothesis
Light-touch mechanotransduction

Modern research confirms that the transfer of mechanical loads to and through biological tissues plays a key role in connective tissue remodeling and the potential therapeutic effects associated with it (Kjær et al. 2009, Humphrey et al. 2014, Ingber et al. 2014). The primary focus regarding this has been on physical activity, tissue engineering and cell behavior, but bodywork as a conduit for mechanotransduction should also be highlighted, with specific techniques presenting different algorithms of mechanical loading (Blyum and Driscoll 2012; Gracovetsky 2016; Chaitow 2018).

"Mechanotransduction is defined as the process by which physical stimulation is converted intracellularly into various types of electrical or chemical signals" (Chiquet et al. 2009). Most research is conducted in vitro by cell biologists, who naturally focus on the mechanosensing aspect: "...how cells sense a mechanical stimulus and convert it into a biochemical, intra-cellular response" (Jansen et al. 2017); but the delivery side of the physical/mechanical stimuli to the human body in vivo remains largely unexplored territory (Gracovetzky 2016).

We can now begin to address this aspect of mechanotransduction via the new bodywork hypothesis through its two essential components, namely, mechanical and physiological. We will address these individually first and then link them together.

I. Mechanics and the stress-strain curve

In bodywork, mechanical stresses are what we deliver manually, and mechanical strains are the body's response to these stresses. The effects of mechanotransduction can be

51

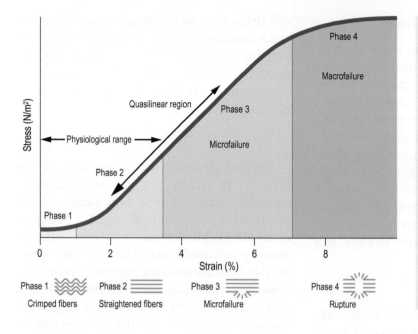

Figure 5.3
The characteristic stress-strain response curve of connective tissues showing four distinct regions (or phases) of changing collagen morphology.

Adapted from Wang (2006).

illustrated by the stress/strain response curve (Kjær et al. 2009) (Figure 5.3).

Figure 5.3 highlights the four phases of collagen morphology in response to external mechanical loads and the corresponding therapeutic hypotheses relevant to the treatment of scar tissue and contractures. It starts with Phase 1, where collagen fibrils have their normal wavy form (labeled as "crimp"), which ensures the tissue's compliance and flexibility that are necessary for the accommodation of our daily movements and postures.

The therapeutic intervention that corresponds to Phase 1 is light massage, where the fiber crimping is maintained and therapeutic benefits are achieved via collateral physical dimensions such as electrical (neurological), hydraulic (circulation and drainage) and heat conduction.

At the other side of the spectrum, Phase 4 is the realm of soft tissue surgery, where the therapeutic intervention hypothesis is the forced mechanical separation of existing collagen bundles followed by restitching at a new length.

Currently prevailing therapeutic intervention hypotheses of body work are largely those of adhesions release or hard self-healing, which assume that the therapeutic effects of manual therapies (including light-touch techniques) belong to the micro-injury/microfailure region of connective tissue strain between 4%-7% (Phase 3).

This hypothesis is very much the legacy of the past when bodywork was forceful, intense and painful, and aimed at enforcing realignment against bodily resistance. However, in the realities of today's light-touch bodywork, the adhesions release hypothesis is highly unrealistic because of the 100-fold mismatch between the minimal magnitude of light touch and force magnitude, which is necessary to induce microfailure within the tightly bonded collagen fibers of a scar/adhesion.

The non-linear-informed bodywork hypothesis (soft self-healing) proposes that the therapeutic effects of light touch on established fibrotic bands stem from the "straightened fibers" region (Phase 2) of the stress-strain curve (where strain is limited to 1%-3%), that is, above the wavy crimp (Phase 1) but below the microfailure adhesions release (Phase 3).

However, expanding our hypothesis towards soft self-healing (Phase 2) is not immediately intuitive because, at first, the Phase 2 significance does not look obvious or meaningful. Apparently the collagen fibers just straighten and nothing structurally transformative appears to happen to them, unlike in Phase 3, where the microscopic failure of collagen bonds makes the structural transformation clear and tangible. In order to

fully appreciate the importance of Phase 2 we need to explore some subtleties.

True linearity, non-linearity, quasilinearity

Figure 5.3 shows the non-linear stress-strain curve with different phases representing the response of living tissues to an imposed mechanical force; but the Phase 2 and 3 regions appear almost to be a straight line and seemingly invite a linear interpretation. This requires clarification!

True linearity does not exist in biology, not even as an approximation. A living system that is so profoundly complex at all its different levels and size-scales (10^{-9}–10^1 m) cannot behave in a linear manner, it is fundamentally impossible.

The entire stress-strain curve is intrinsically non-linear, and although the Phase 2 and 3 parts of the stress-strain curve appear to be linear, they are in fact double non-linear.

"To promote mechanical homeostasis in health, cells must use negative feedback mechanisms that sense changes within the extracellular matrix (ECM) and restore values back towards normal [Figure 5.4]. For example, acute *increases* in stiffness should trigger mechanisms that render the ECM more compliant, whereas acute *decreases* in stiffness should trigger pathways that result in stiffening" (Humphrey et al. 2014).

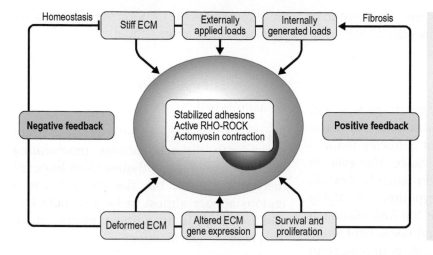

Figure 5.4
Negative feedback mechanisms restoring normal mechanical properties of ECM.

Reproduced from Humphrey et al. (2014).

Thanks to these two intrinsic non-linearities, which are powered by negative feedback mechanisms within the ECM, the extrinsic double non-linear outcome of the stress-strain curve is kept at its lowest during Phases 2 and 3, creating an outcome that looks linear but is intrinsically controlled by the built-in non-linearities of mechanical homeostasis.

In order to find the terminology that reflects the different grades of non-linearity, it makes sense to borrow a distinction that Benoit Mandelbrot (the author of *fractal theory*) applied to the classification of randomness. Standard discourse at that time held randomness and regularity apart while Mandelbrot (2004) highlighted that randomness was fundamental and everywhere; it just had a different intensity and behavior. In other words, the processes which appear externally regular are still internally underpinned by randomness. The regularity assumption is thus fundamentally misleading and not applicable anywhere, although it is mathematically convenient. He addressed this challenge by introducing the concepts of wild and mild randomness, replacing the original dichotomy of "randomness" and "regularity" with the fundamentally consistent approach, where the "regularity" equals mild randomness.

Biomechanics is in a similar conundrum. Linear assumptions are endorsed because they are convenient for calculations, but unfortunately this convenience leads to false conclusions on the linear behavior of tissue instead of looking for a more accurate understanding of the essence of biological non-linearity.

Following Mandelbrot's template, we can apply the similar distinction of wild and mild non-linearity to the effects of mechanotransduction on biological tissues.

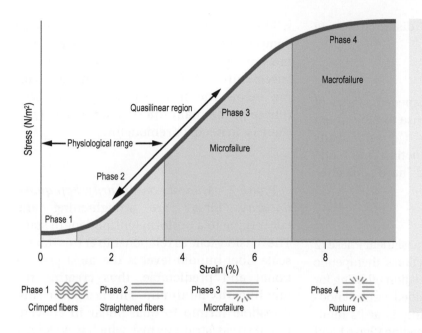

Figure 5.5
The stress-strain response curve highlighting the combined quasilinear region of Phases 2 and 3.

Wild and mild non-linearity

Non-linearity is a very broad term that has many facets, but for our current practical purposes it is sufficient to focus on the disproportionality/unpredictability aspect of non-linearity, examining the relationship between the ways in which the increments of stress impact convert into the increments of strain response.

The more disproportionate and unpredictable the impact-response relationship then the wilder the non-linearity; conversely, the more proportional and predictable it is then the milder the non-linearity.

Let's look at the stress-strain curve phases through this lens (Figure 5.5).

Natural movement in living bodies is accommodated by tissue crimp (Phase 1 of the stress/strain curve). This is a wild non-linearity, where impact/response ratios are irregular, unpredictable and incalculable. However, these accommodations occur within the safe range and do not trigger the dual negative feedback mechanisms.

Phases 2 and 3 are mildly non-linear because the stress-strain and tension-length relationship within those ranges exhibit much less irregularity and unpredictability in their impact-response thanks to the dual negative feedback mechanisms of stiffness and compliance within the ECM.

At Phase 4, non-linearity becomes wild again because the impact-response relationship jumps to being extremely disproportionate and unpredictable.

In order to reflect the special status of Phases 2 and 3 it makes sense to label them collectively as "quasilinear" ("quasi" means "as if") with a further distinction into "soft" quasilinearity (Phase 2) and "hard" quasilinearity (Phase 3).

These mildly non-linear/quasilinear Phases 2 and 3 are mechanotransduction's therapeutic impact window, a special situation allowing for somewhat predictable and guided tissue remodeling because the non-linearity is at its minimum compared with the preceding Phase 1 and also following Phase 4. Which therapy window is more promising? Historically, both scientific biomechanics and bodywork therapists alike have chosen to focus on Phase 3.

Nowadays, 21st century scientists invite us to embrace the less obvious Phase 2 by shifting our focus to threshold events and phase transitions. Such a change of emphasis is information-centric: How valuable and how accurate is the remodeling information at each of the phases?

Phase transitions

<u>Phase 1</u> – Crimp. *Wild non-linearity*. At this wavy phase the collagen fibers have lots of spare length, thus making the microscale tension/length relationships for fascia/fibers incalculable and maximizing the non-linear wildness. This is normal non-linear tissue compliance within everyday macroscale movements and mobility. When tissues successfully conform to mechanical loading below the threshold of quasilinearity (Phase 2) the main information is positive – there is no need for remodeling.

<u>Phase 2</u> – *Mildest non-linearity. Soft quasilinearity*. Fibers are straightening and converging to a uniform tension-length state. The tension-length relationship at this microscale fiber-bundle level is the most proportional and predictable, thus creating the non-linearity minimum. This is a phase shift threshold (crimp to quasilinear in conventional stress/strain terms), which is no longer a movement but an almost uniform (quasi-static) strain-energy (SE) state. Dual negative feedback mechanisms balancing stiffness and compliance within ECM can then work with most accuracy.

<u>Phase 3</u> – *Mild non-linearity. Hard quasilinearity*. Fibers at microscale experience microfailure at variable rates and lengths and, as a result, the intrinsic tension-length relationships within the fiber-bundles become more irregular and unpredictable. With larger stresses the number of microfailures grows and overall non-uniformity escalates. Additional protective data (pain, etc.) impacts the tension parameter and the error rate grows. Overall, non-linearity is still much milder than at Phases 1 and 4 but it increases dramatically compared with Phase 2, while the accuracy of remodeling information falls down.

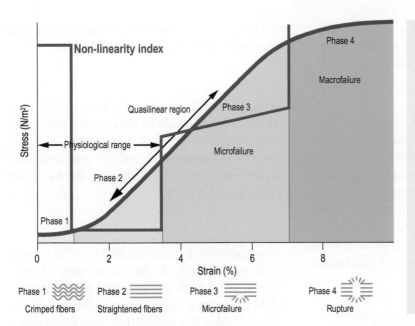

Phase 1 〰〰 Crimped fibers
Phase 2 ═══ Straightened fibers
Phase 3 ⫶⫶ Microfailure
Phase 4 ☀ Rupture

Figure 5.6
The non-linearity index illustrating the wilder and milder unpredictability in tension-length relationships underpinning the stress-strain curve.

Summary: Non-linear-informed light-touch bodywork hypothesis formulated compactly

For non-linear biological tissues, the light-touch induced transition from Phase 1 to Phase 2 is the most important mechanotransduction phase transition (Figure 5.6):

(a) It is the very first phase transition of the stress/strain curves – from tension-length incomputable wild non-linearity to computable mild/ soft quasilinearity – hence the most informative threshold effect.

Threshold effects are the causative factors/triggers of phase transitions. For example, ice formation from liquid water is a phase transition that is triggered by the threshold effects related to the nucleation of crystals within the previously liquid water. Depending on

factors like impurities, pressure and flow, such a phase transition might happen at different temperatures in the vicinity of 0 degrees Celsius.

(b) At Phase 2 the soft self-healing is the most accurate, having a minimal error rate because the system is at its minimal non-linearity index thus being the least irregular/unpredictable and the most controllable.

(c) Manually, the threshold effects of Phase 1 to Phase 2 transitions are precision-based and not force magnitude-based, hence minimal light-touch forces are sufficient, making a 100-fold super-effectiveness claim plausible.

Let us link it with real bodywork experiences. How do we describe when a good light-touch therapist delivers proper initial manual contact: light hands, feather touch, soft entry, smooth transition, etc.? What are these experiences? Phase 1 to Phase 2 transitions.

Such manual guidance is more than common language, it is an algorithmic/ operational description which instructs a therapist how to achieve phase transitions through threshold effects and optimization criteria in respect to Phases 1, 2 and 3. These are the logical equations that bodyworkers solve in every single therapy session! Threshold effects characterize the phase transitions.

II. Physiology: soft self-healing versus hard self-healing

After seeing the leading importance of Phase 2 in the mechanical effects of mechanotransduction on connective tissue, let us explore Phase 2 physiology, beginning with a direct question: What does it take to achieve at least partial reversibility of established scar tissue? Where exactly does it happen? What processes should be activated? What internal agents are capable of such remodeling? Modern research answers clearly (see below).

ECM remodeling

Remodeling occurs within the ECM. "ECM is a diverse collection of proteins and sugars surrounding cells in all solid tissues; mainly composed of an interlocking mesh of fibrillar and non-fibrillar collagens; elastic fibers; glycosaminoglycan (GAG)-containing non-

collagenous glycoproteins (hyaluronan and proteoglycans)" (Cox and Erler 2011).

ECM provides a structural scaffold upon which cells grow, differentiate, organize and function. The ECM of bones and connective tissues bears most of the physical load acting on our body (Chiquet et al. 2009; Tschumperlin 2015).

Is it possible to remodel ECM and to reverse once-established ECM structure? Fortunately, yes. "Both the proteins and sugars of ECM undergo a mechano-regulation process that includes the deposition, rearrangement, or removal of matrix to maintain overall form and function" (Humphrey et al. 2014, Chiquet et al. 2009).

What are the internal agents of ECM structural maintenance and renewal? The fibroblasts are considered the key players in ECM maintenance and adaptation to changes in homeostasis and remodeling (Kjaer et al. 2009, Tschumperlin 2015).

Motivated fibroblast networks

So far so good. We have solid proof that fibroblast activity within the ECM has an immense remodeling and structural reversibility capacity in self-healing mode. But where is the tipping point? Why does the regenerative self-healing sometimes take place but at other times not? How can we tap into this remodeling capacity of the fibroblasts in a systematic, predictable and guided way?

One obvious avenue is the micro-injury domain of Phase 3, which triggers the chemical signaling that mobilizes the fibroblasts into hard self-healing with forced emergency remodeling that originates from the micro-damage site (Li et al. 2019).

Within the field of soft, light-touch bodywork we have a different interest, that is, does research indicate more ecological soft self-healing ways that are Phase 2-compatible and avoid micro-damage to tissues? Exploring this path requires a closer look at the fibroblast "families" because apparently not all of them participate equally in remodeling. Li et al. (2019) introduces an elegant term, describing the fibroblasts which actively remodel the ECM as being "motivated" (the passive ones are "dormant").

While the internal filamentous cytoskeletons of active fibroblasts are tensionally linked with each other through transmembranous proteins and fibers within the ECM, the dormant ones float in suspension and assume a more rounded cellular shape (Langevin et al. 2004; Kjaer 2009; Ingber et al. 2014). Langevin et al. (2004) bring further insight: "...fibroblasts are not separate cells, but are linked together in a reticular network extending throughout the whole body."

This understanding is helpful in our quest for Phase 2 remodeling, indicating that soft self-healing has to provide proper mechanical cues which maximize the number of motivated members within a regional fibroblast family.

III. Mechanics and physiology, biotensegrity

To bring together the mechanics and physiology of Phase 2 mechanotransduction requires us to answer two main questions: "How does Phase 2 mechanotransduction 'motivate' the fibroblasts?" and "What specific ECM remodeling instructions does Phase 2 induce?"

Fortunately, solutions to both of these questions have a common root. What looked like a disadvantage of Phase 2 at the intuitive level – its uniformity where nothing special happens/just straightening of collagen fibers – now becomes the major advantage! In essence, "the straightening of the fibers under tension" at Phase 2 means that tissues undergo a uniform deformation characterized by a uniform strain energy (SE) density that creates a uniform strain-field. Such phenomena are studied extensively by new complexity sciences, namely, peridynamics, uniform deformation theory, mesomechanics and nucleation theory.

How does Phase 2 influence the networked fibroblasts?

The co-existence of the motivated (tension-engaged/high strain) fibroblasts and dormant (tension-disengaged/low strain) fibroblasts is the equivalent of the metastable mechanical equilibrium, where the high and low strain areas are locked within their respective phase boundaries (Dayal and Bhattacharya 2006, Silling and Lehoucq 2010, Kalikmanov 2013, Silling 2018).

Phase 2 uniform deformation allows the SE to exchange between the high and low strain regions and to eventually settle at a new minimum. Consequently, areas that were previously locked in SE imbalance can now integrate into a new, more balanced state with the excess SE (previously phase boundary-locked) dissipating. It is thus safe to assume that this SE redistribution occurs when light-touch practitioners experience sensations of "melting tense tissues" and "adhesions release". From the perspective of 21st century complexity science, these experiences are most likely reflecting Phase 2 rather than Phase 3 effects.

What specific ECM remodeling instructions does Phase 2 induce?

Fibroblasts form two classes of network coupling: fibroblast-to-fibroblast and fibroblast-to-ECM.

First, Phase 2-induced SE redistribution allows the fibroblast-to-fibroblast network to rearrange itself into a better long-term balance (regional minimum SE) that is likely to reduce the overloading of highly motivated fibroblasts while bringing the dormant ones out of hibernation. As a result, new

tension lines within the cytoskeletal filament networks are likely to be formed.

Second, it then becomes logical to assume that the SE-induced redistribution of tension lines and new activity within the fibroblast-to-fibroblast network leads to the corresponding remodeling of the fibroblasts-to-ECM connections and a new improved state that follows the same internal SE minimization criteria. "Strain rather than stress/torque determines the collagen-synthesis stimulating response" (Kjær et al. 2009).

These two compact answers are the essence of the SE phase boundaries reset hypothesis, that is, the non-linearity-informed light-touch bodywork hypothesis (or the soft self-healing hypothesis). They finally allow us to address the premise with which we started this chapter, concerning the unreasonable effectiveness of light touch.

Phase 3 micro-injury adhesions release interpretation was tightly pegged to force magnitude. The light touch delivers only one hundredth of this, which is too little to break collagen bundles. This mismatch made light touch appear unreasonable and unscientific.

The non-linearity-informed approach points out that the lead factor in remodeling is not the force magnitude but the force density (the force per unit volume). What matters for the reset of phase boundaries between the motivated (high strain) and dormant (low strain) fibroblast and ECM regions is the uniformity of the SE density, that is, quality not quantity. Phase 2 mechanotransduction operates at low force magnitudes but provides the uniformity of the deformation field thus making the light touch perfectly reasonable. QED.

Conclusion: Phase 2 mechanotransduction and biotensegrity

The new complexity sciences of peridynamics, mesomechanics and nucleation theory are heavily mathematical, thus making them difficult for most bodyworkers to draw on for practical guidance.

Fortunately, this problem is resolved by biotensegrity, a vector geometry perspective which combines the same conclusions with intuitive understanding and experiential 3D models.

The main features and applications of biotensegrity are extensively covered throughout this book, and therefore a brief review of how biotensegrity corresponds to Phase 2 mechanotransduction will suffice. Indeed, the answer is provided in the name. "Tensegrity" stands for tensional integrity, which in a compact form combines the properties just discussed in the SE phase boundaries reset hypothesis.

- Tensional – indicates the focus on the SE fields.
- Integrity – highlights the network integration of all the elements.
- Tensional integrity range – this points to the region within the networked tensional system where the uniform deformation field spreads from local to regional to global, and vice versa.

In brief, biotensegrity points directly to Phase 2 mechanotransduction that spreads from an area of contact to a uniform deformation throughout the entire networked system, as opposed to the accumulation of local discontinuous strains of Phase 3.

This makes biotensegrity a source of essential guidance for bodyworkers, suggesting the following core algorithm: Wherever there is an imbalance and discontinuity within the soft tissues – blend carefully into those during your treatment; meet their surface tension without distortions; connect to the surrounding areas for broader tensional integration; gently nudge and – just stay with it, thus allowing the self-organizing magic of SE redistribution to do its work!

Light-touch practice already delivers fantastic results – when we are essentially intuitive empiricists who are fragmented among proprietary therapies. However, the history of other professions shows that we can gain collectively by embracing a united bodywork approach, recognizing our commonalities ahead of our differences (Gracovetsky 2016). This has the potential to give us better guidance, a better sharing of experiences, improved communication with other health practitioners and, most importantly, a shorter path to new discoveries and therapy protocols.

A bodywork hypothesis is never going to be final: it should always be a work in progress where we continually strive for improvement. A non-linearity-informed light-touch bodywork hypothesis is intended to be a step in this direction, helping us to recognize our commonalities and to reach out to the larger world of 21st century science.

References

Barnes, M. P., and Johnson, G. R. (2008). *Upper motor neurone syndrome and spasticity.* Cambridge, UK: Cambridge University Press.

Blyum, L., and Driscoll, M. (2012). Mechanical stress transfer – the fundamental physical basis of all manual therapy techniques. *Journal of Bodywork & Movement Therapies.* 16:520–527.

Chaitow, L. (2018). Fascial well-being: Mechanotransduction in manual and movement therapies. *Journal of Bodywork & Movement Therapies.* 22:235–236.

Chiquet, M., Gelman, L., Lutz, R., and Maier, S. (2009). From mechanotransduction to extracellular matrix gene expression in fibroblasts. *Biochimica et Biophysica Acta.* 1793:911–920.

Cox, T., and Erler, J. T. (2011). Remodeling and homeostasis of the extracellular matrix: implications for fibrotic diseases and cancer. *Disease Models & Mechanisms.* 4:165–178.

Dayal, D., and Bhattacharya, K. (2006) Kinetics of phase transformations in the peridynamics formulation of continuum mechanics. *Journal of the Mechanics and Physics of Solids*, 54(9), pp. 1811–1842.

Gracovetsky, S. (2016). Can fascia's characteristics be influenced by manual therapy? *Journal of Bodywork & Movement Therapies.* 20:893–897.

Humphrey, J. D., Dufresne, E. R., and Schwartz, M. A. (2014). Mechanotransduction and extracellular matrix homeostasis. *Nature Reviews Molecular and Cell Biology.* 15:802–812.

Ingber, D. E., Wang, N., and Stamenović, D. (2014). Tensegrity, cellular biophysics, and the mechanics of living systems. *Reports on Progress in Physics.* 77:046603.

Jansen, K. A., Atherton, P., and Ballestrem, C. (2017). Mechanotransduction at the cell-matrix interface. *Seminars in Cell and Developmental Biology.* 71:75–83.

Kalikmanov, V. I. (2013). *Nucleation Theory. Series: Lecture Notes in Physics* (volume 860). Springer.

Kjaer, M., Langberg, H., Heinemeier, K., Bayer, M. L., Hansen, M., Holm, L., Doessing, L., Kongsgaard, M., Krogsgaard, M. R., and Magnusson, S. R. (2009). From mechanical loading to collagen synthesis, structural changes and function in human tendon. *Scandinavian Journal of Medical Science and Sports*. 19:500–510.

Langevin, H., Cornbrooks, C., and Taatjes, D. (2004). Fibroblasts form a body-wide cellular network. *Histochemistry and Cell Biology*. 122:7–15.

Li, Y., Xiao, Z., Zhou, Y., Zheng, S., An, Y., Huang, W., He, H., Yang, Y., Li, S., Chen, Y., Xiao, J., and Wu, J. (2019). Controlling multiscale network structure of fibers to stimulate wound matrix rebuilding by fibroblast differentiation. *ACS Applied Materials and Interfaces*. 11:28377–28386.

Mandelbrot, B., and Hudson, R. L. (2004). *The (Mis)behavior of Markets: A Fractal View of Financial Turbulence*. New York, NY: Basic Books.

Silling, S. A. (2018). Modeling microstructure and defects with peridynamics. *SIAM Conference on Mathematical Aspects of Materials Science*. Portland, OR, 11 July 2018.

Silling, S. A., and Lehoucq, R. B. (2010). Peridynamic theory of solid mechanics. *Advances in Applied Mechanics*. 44:73–168.

Tschumperlin, D. (2015). Matrix, Mesenchyme, and Mechanotransduction. *Annals of the American Thoracic Society*. 12:S24–S29.

Wang, J. (2006). Mechanobiology of tendon. *Journal of Biomechanics*. 39:1563–1582.

Wigner, E. (1960). The unreasonable effectiveness of mathematics in the natural sciences Communications. *Pure and Applied Mathematics*. XIII:1–14.

A clinical anatomist's experience of scars and adhesions in the cadaver

Chapter 6

John Sharkey

Introduction

A clinical anatomist provides educational training involving cadaveric dissection to undergraduate medical students, post-graduate medical specialists (i.e., surgeons, anesthetists, gynecologists) and a wide range of professionals expressing an interest in human anatomy. Historically, the emphasis of anatomical study has been on "where?" Where is the superior mesenteric artery? Where is the suspensory muscle of the duodenum (or the ligament of Treitz)? Where is Meckel's cave? Where does the phrenic nerve arise and where is its anatomical path? The clinical anatomist thrives on detail and precision, for example, identifying and describing embryologically informed fascial entry points for surgical interventions in an effort to ensure minimally invasive surgery.

Unfortunately, the oft-used phrase "minimally invasive surgery" can be a misleading idiom, giving a false sense of security to all of those involved. Knowledge coming from biotensegrity-focused dissection provides a unique educational experience whereby we can better appreciate the inner reality of our soft matter architecture, our continuity and our connectedness.

As a clinical anatomist, working with human cadavers for more than 30 years, I am accustomed to finding adhesions and scars throughout the remains of donors.

Some scars and adhesions are accompanied by surface reflections that provide an immediate visual alert to the likely process under which the scar occurred (such as degloving, burns, post-operative, post-traumatic, atrophic, post-infective or diabetic wound scars), providing the possibility of expectation concerning what lies beneath the insult. It is also possible to discover adhesions deep to uninjured skin, skin that does not reflect such insults.

In such cases, one finds evidence in the deeper fascia and related connective tissues reflecting sequelae of a pathological condition, atrophy or illness (Figure 6.1). Incision-related scars and the fibrotic, hard, dense tissues resulting from surgery can have a negative effect on movement and health.

There is currently a dearth of data in the literature regarding the topic of scars, adhesions and the cadaveric experience.

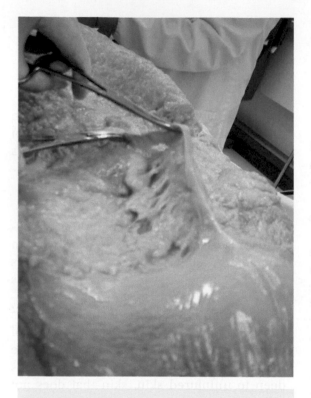

Figure 6.1
Thickened, densified scar tissue runs from the dermis down to the deepest fascia profunda.

Image: J. Sharkey, 2017.

This chapter provides the observational findings of dissection investigations in an effort to postulate the environments, settings and surroundings required to ensure the health and functionality of the connective tissues generally, and fascia specifically. The introduction of Thiel soft-fixed cadavers, supported by learning outcomes derived from the dissection of fresh frozen cadaveric specimens, has enabled fascial tissues and related structures to be investigated in a way which was not possible with more traditional fixative solutions such as formalin and formaldehyde.

Fascial anatomy and its classification into functional hierarchical categories

The Thiel dissection experience has given unique insights into fascial anatomy and has led to the classification of fascia into functional hierarchical categories, which include gliding (see Figure 6.2), restraining, containing, force-transductive, communicative, septal, invaginating and osseous. The terms "loose" and "areolar" are avoided in this context because they embrace and relate to all of the classifications of fascial tissue.

While fascia is literally everywhere, its morphology changes specific to the forces influencing and informing its construct. Fascia-making cells (fibroblasts) respond to changes in tension and compression resulting in a functionally responsive connective tissue that facilitates what is required in a specific location. Changes in forces generated within or acting upon specific anatomical locations have local and wider reaching implications. Such implications result in over- or under-stimulation of cellular activity, leading to weakened structures, sticky or immobile tissues, densification (or hypertrophy), thinning (or atrophy), excessive compression, or tension, resulting in inappropriate, energy-demanding (i.e., non-economical) motion and pain (Pavan et al. 2014).

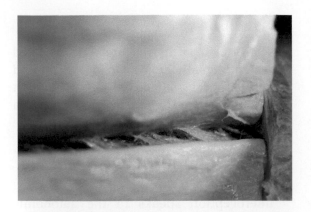

Figure 6.2
The gliding of structures relative to each other is supported by appropriate levels of hyaluronic acid and the freedom of shared, continuous inter-planary fascial structures to change shape by elongating (unwinding) or compressing (winding) in a telescopic manner where no individual molecule, organelle, cell or fiber is truly shortening or lengthening.

Gliding

Gliding means to pass imperceptibly, to move smoothly and continuously along, as if without effort or resistance (see Figure 6.2). Connective tissue has no layers, only continuity and densification with specialization along a continuum. Layers are a man-made construct useful in situations such as surgery, dissection and ultrasonography. Fascia, specifically, thins and thickens from superficial (i.e. surface) to deep. In keeping with Newton's third law[1], moving the skin in one direction will result in tissue deep to the skin moving in the opposite direction. Tissue deeper to that tissue will also move in an oppo-

site direction and so on, down to the deepest tissues. If the tissue is healthy there will be no "sliding". Sliding involves continuous contact between two surfaces that results in friction. Friction creates heat, irritating and breaking the integrity of tissue, causing inflammation, swelling, loss of motion, and eventually pain. Gliding allows for frictionless movement of tissues of relative density and depth (see Figure 6.2).

Restraining

Healthy skin ligaments, or retinacula, are examples of tissues which have a specific limit to their ability to shape change. This physiological limit provides deceleration of movement in a body part or segment in an effort to restrain or constrain stretching and ensure integrity. Stretchmarks on the abdomens of post-pregnant women are evidence of the morphological changes skin is subjected to when the restraining retinacula are truly lengthened, never to return to offer their restraining capability.

Containing

Readers should be aware that fasciae act as a conduit containing and enclosing blood vessels, nerves, interstitium and lymphatic tissues that are integral to optimal health (Figure 6.3). One can immediately appreciate the multiple impacts on force transmission, physiology and metabolism, both locally and more globally, when fascia has morphologically become disorganized, densified, fibrosed and immobile. It is well established that

---

1 For every action, there is an equal and opposite reaction.

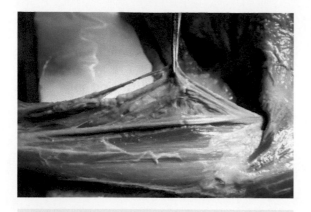

Figure 6.3
Fascia contains nerves, blood vessels and other important anatomical structures necessary for health and well-being.

Image: J. Sharkey, 2018.

scar tissue can negatively inform complex molecular and cellular interactions while the body attempts to heal and recover (Fitch and Silver 2008). Fascia such as perimysium provides containment to bundles of muscle fibers and, in the event of damage caused by internal or external forces, that damage is restricted to the most minimal surface area.

Force-transductive

Fascia acts to facilitate the exchange of mechanical forces, translating those forces locally and globally (including via the skeletal system) into cell-specific molecular pathways (Purslow 2010, Sharkey 2017). Forces of compression and tension are essential for cellular activity, ensuring that mechanical forces are translated into metabolism and physiology.

Communicative

Fascia is rich with free and encapsulated nerve endings, including Golgi, Ruffini and Pacini corpuscles (Stecco et al. 2007). What is less appreciated is the role of fascia as a communicator of emotion, providing a bridge between interoception and exteroception.

Interoception speaks to the autonomic and medullar homoeostatic centers, the brain stem, the frontal cingulate cortex and dorsal posterior insula, via the thalamocortical circuit. Interoception can modulate the exteroceptive representation of the body, while setting parameters concerning pain tolerance. Structural changes in the connective tissues, such as scarring, fibrosis and adhesions, may dysregulate the pathways which are responsible for providing details regarding the status of our structural state, and could therefore cause a distortion of one's body image (Tsay et al. 2015).

Septal

Fascia is continuous and ubiquitous, wrapping up or surrounding, investing and interpenetrating structures, and providing a partition that separates yet forms an integral aspect of the continuity of our form. Septa can include muscle envelopes, joint capsules, organ capsules and retinacula. Also, fascia can thicken to provide an intermediate partition between muscles or individual muscle fibers. Delving deeper to the micro-level, septa can be found in the form of membranes, allowing a delineation between two virtual spaces.

Gross examples include the ventricular septa separating the right and left ventricles or the intermuscular septa providing both autonomy and synergy between muscles, such as the lateral raphe.

Invaginating

An example of the many invaginations in embryonic development is the processus vaginalis, an outcome of the descent of the testis from the innermost parietal peritoneum. Invaginating tissue results in both a reinforcing and thickening of the fascia, and consequently specific anatomical regions can become thinner and weaker, usually at the distal or proximal portions. This can predispose the tissue to an increased risk of herniation.

Osseous

Fascia is connective tissue. Connective tissue is continuous throughout the human form. Coming to terms with continuity can be a challenge. The vocabulary used to describe human architecture can create a misleading disconnect that is man-made. It could be argued that connective tissues that are not considered fascia are internally external to the fascia. Bone is internally internal (keep in mind that this is a language of convenience, as everything deep to the skin is internal). According to Levin (2018), "If fascia is considered a continuum, and tendons and ligaments are fascia, then to what do they continue when they transition to bone? The tendon at one end of a muscle is a continuum of the fascia components of the muscle and continuous with the tendon on the other end of the muscle. If tendons and ligaments are continuations of the muscle fascia, then the periosteum (fascia by everyone's definition) is a continuation (not an attachment but a continuation) of the tendons, the Sharpey's fibers are a continuation of the periosteum and the fibrous matrix of the bone is a continuation of Sharpey's fibers and out the other side. The bone's fascia interpenetrates the bone as the muscle's fascia interpenetrates muscle. Bone is not a crystalline column of calcium; it is a stiffly starched shirt very much dependent on the structure of its fabric for both form and function."

The pervasive fascial tissue system

The pervasive fascial tissue system is not a perfect construct in evolutionary terms. Even without consideration of surgical interventions and the resulting negative impact of weakening fascial structures, fascia has site-specific anatomical areas which have an increased risk of tearing or insult due to the thinner nature of their connective tissue construct. Examples of this include the epigastric region due to a single sheet of fascia, in contrast to a more robust double sheet of fascia in other abdominal areas. The "floor" of the inguinal canal or the superficial inguinal ring (Hesselbach's fascia), as well as the femoral canal, are other examples. The arcuate line represents a transitional point in the fascia from thick, strong connective tissue to a thin, weaker tissue. It is at this anatomical position, located at the lower or inferior lateral margin of rectus sheath, where Spigelian hernias (although rare) can present. Surgery also weakens the fascia (Figure 6.4) and damages its integrity, while the resulting

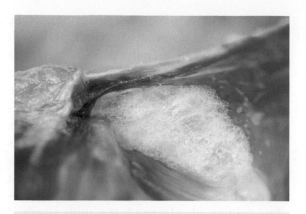

Figure 6.4
"Pulling" or "lifting" connective tissues, including muscles, disrupts the mechanical construct of the gliding planes, creating emergent architecture resembling a thickened web-like or cotton candy structure. Once disrupted, this tissue plane will house fibrotic, scarred, dehydrated and immobile tissue.

excessive pulling forces of the scarred tissues draw and collect the connective tissue, sucking the associated neural, vascular, lymphatic and fluid structures (and associated osseous assemblies) into itself.

Physiology creates heat in our body through the breakdown of adenosine triphosphate. Body heat should not be created via friction. Friction occurs when there is pathology in the body. As a consequence of scarring, changes in tension and compression reduce the critical fiber distance among muscular entities. Fascial septa are impeded. Immobile, compressed structures create friction in what would otherwise be a frictionless plain. Irritated tissue planes result in a subsequent inflammatory response, swelling, edema, ecchymosis, increased levels of hyaluronic and lactic acid, reduced gliding, and a disruption to effective local and body-wide force transmission (Figure 6.2).

Variation is the norm

Through the study of anatomy via dissection we appreciate that variation is the norm, with no two bodies ever quite the same. The cartoon-like illustrations provided in anatomy textbooks that show attachment sites, nerve branches and other aspects of anatomical structures are far removed from the reality witnessed in dissection. A false appreciation of our soft tissue architecture due to the simplification of muscle fibers, which are described without mention of their surrounding investing fabric, the myofascia, and the many roles it plays based on its three-dimensional continuity, has promoted a misrepresentation of our connected self (Figure 6.5).

The fertile sensory innervation of fascia

In 1957, Stillwell confirmed the fertile sensory innervation of fascia, confirmed as having as many as 10-fold more sensory receptors in the fascial tissues compared with muscles (Stillwell 1957). In 2016, Grunwald updated this figure in his book, *Homo hapticus*, estimating that there are 100 million receptors in the body-wide fascial system (Grunwald 2016). The true disruption of the connective tissues and their associated neurovascular and lymphatic vessels, occurring as a consequence

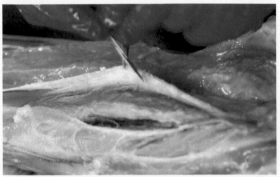

Figure 6.5
View of the muscle fiber and its surrounding fascial fabric.

Image: J. Sharkey, 2018.

of surgical intervention deep to the skin, is not always immediately evident based on the surface markings left by the surgical entry point(s) or incisions made upon the skin.

Minimally invasive surgery is akin to saying that during a war one country minimally invades another. While a surgeon's intention is to reduce (as much as possible) the disruption to a patient's tissues and amount of post-operative pain, the reality is that, regardless of the evidence left on the surface of the skin, an iceberg develops in the dermis, hypodermis and deeper in the fascial depths, often embracing the sandy shoreline of bone (Figure 6.6). Such impacts are greatly influenced by the age, health and gender of the patient. Adhered and fibrotic tissue will now call for the establishment of new neuromuscular strategies to accomplish any given movement.

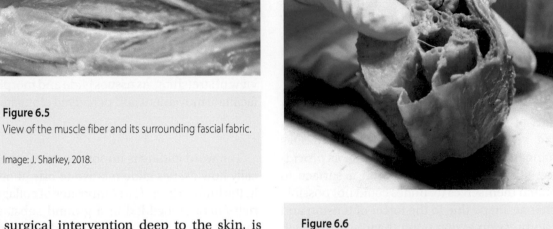

Figure 6.6
The fascial net relationship continuous with the sandy shores of the bone. Having removed the muscle fibers (and associated endomysial fascia), one has a visual context in which to place a new appreciation of continuity and force transfer.

Image: Stecco, C., Sharkey, J., Schleip, R. (2018). Human Fascial Net Plastination Project.

No research, only a suggestion for research

Figure 6.5 shows a clear incision having been made to the superficial aspect of the fascia profunda (with the skin and superficial fascia reflected), including a disruption to the epimysium surrounding and investing the muscle gaster. This fascial tissue would be best considered as osseofascial tissue, therefore taking into consideration the vital, embryological continuity with the bones. When I was growing up, adults often said that children should be seen and not heard. Thankfully this is not the case these days; however, for the application of this analogy, the bones are seen as children by too many professionals whose training did not encourage them to consider (or pay much attention to) bone. Continuing this analogy, the bones are neither seen nor heard (unless there is a bone break). The general view of bone is that it is considered to be hard, unyielding, stiff tissue, and not an integral part of the fascial system. Bone is viewed as the scaffolding that our myofascial tissues hang from. The role of bone is seen as providing our contractile tissues with a surface to attach themselves to. Bones could not possibly change shape due to the forces of tension and compression acting upon them (e.g., through impacts). Or could they?

Before the emergence of a substantial amount of research informing us that fascia should be given more consideration than it was previously, for the most part we were ignorant of the vital role which fascia plays as the main tissue of communication, interoception, proprioception, slow contraction, posture and pain, plus others. Similarly, I propose that not only does bone shorten, rotate, side-bend and lengthen (or unwind) short of fracture, it is also a major contributor in storing and returning forces that we have hitherto attributed almost exclusively to tendons and muscle fibers.

This is an important consideration when working with scar tissue. Scars can be worked

from the inside out, working purposefully and specifically with the bone and, where applicable, the inter-osseous membranes.

Visible everywhere are structures that ensure a gliding movement between the aponeuroses, the fatty fascial structures with their associated fascial laminae and the dermis. This has implications regarding our view of stretching, as tissues glide and morph to facilitate movement and perceived elongation.

The word gliding is important here, specifically how tissues glide relative to one another in the human body (as composites of collagen-rich fibers embedded in a ground substance matrix). However, they do not *slide* relative to each other unless there is pathology such as scarring or adhesions. Sliding would result in friction. Friction would cause excessive heat and cause further tissue irritation leading to sustained inflammation and a consequential inflammatory response. When working optimally, biotensegrity structures are frictionless, as can be observed in the joints of the body.

Figure 6.7 shows continuous adaptive vacuolar structures emerging from the supportive fascial network. This emerging vacuolar structure, exposed by fresh frozen dissection, has very interesting capabilities. It is able to change shape when tension is applied and, after the tension is removed, to return to its original state while continuing to maintain the same volume. "The presence of a vacuolar system in the fascia provides a stable, yet flexible environment necessary for fascia

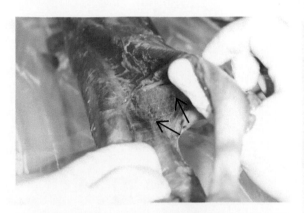

Figure 6.7
A fresh frozen cadaver specimen of an anterior forearm. The arrows point to the continuous adaptive vacuolar structures emerging from the supportive fascial network.

Image: J. Sharkey, 2010.

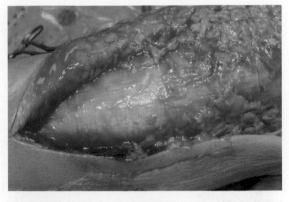

Figure 6.8
One can visualize the disrupting insults to skin and deeper connective tissues, the result of surgical incisions, leading to loss of integrity as a result of inevitable compositional changes.

Image: J. Sharkey, 2010.

to act as a force and tension transmitter" (Huijing 2009).

Direction-reliant, biomechanical behavior of skin is significantly impacted by the structural orientation of its collagen-rich fibrous network and its viscous ground substance matrix. Disrupting insults to skin (i.e., skin injuries), such as those resulting from surgical incisions, lead to superficial and deeper structural changes in the connective tissues (see Figure 6.8) and loss of integrity as a result of inevitable compositional changes (Tabibian et al. 2017).

The likelihood of adhesions, densification and reduced pliability is greatest in the

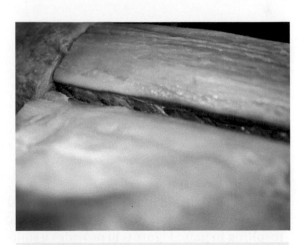

Figure 6.9
The likelihood of adhesions, densification and reduced pliability is greatest in the connective tissue interfaces, leading to reduced movement quality and the inevitability of pathological changes resulting in pain.

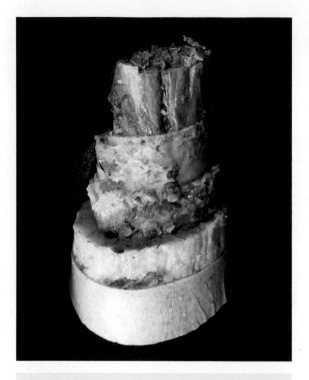

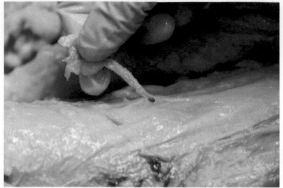

Figure 6.11

The deep fascial wrapping (often referred to as a bag) acting as a septum, a gliding surface and, interestingly, as a conduit for neurovasuclar structures. Here, we see a neurovascular structure penetrate the fascia rising from the depths. One can visualize how constriction at this juncture due to scarring would have a dramatic effect upon neural and vascular activity.

Image: J. Sharkey, 2018.

Figure 6.10

A staircase visual representation showing the skin (as surface) connecting the deep fascia to the undersurface of the integument.

Image: Stecco, C., Sharkey, J., Schleip, R. (2018). Human Fascial Net Plastination Project.

connective tissue interfaces (Figure 6.9), leading to reduced movement quality and the inevitability of pathological changes, resulting in pain. Figure 6.10 provides a staircase visual representation showing the skin (as surface), with the next morphological change at the depth of the superficial adipose tissue containing fat lobules and strong retinacula (or skin ligaments), connecting the deep fascia to the undersurface of the integument. The deep fascia surrounds and penetrates the muscle, nerves, blood vessels, and eventually ligaments. Therapists can appreciate how forces generated by the muscle fibers act upon the osseofascial system tensioning the bones to move, while also stiffening joints and specific myokinetic chains. Importantly, biotensegrity-focused dissection demonstrates how the myofascia provides structural integrity affecting blood supply, venous return and neural entrapment (see Figure 6.11). Dense, fibrotic fascia stifles the gliding relationships of superficial to deeper structures resulting in tethered tissues, and possibly pain.

Neural and vascular changes to the architecture that are comprehensive and global have been regularly identified in cadaveric dissection. The scar that forms at the surface of the skin will typically fashion itself along the same route and course as the incision, resulting in a set of new anatomical and physiological changes. These morphological changes now command and dictate the vector and orientation of the scar tissue collagen net and the deeper mucopolysaccharide ground substance. Such morphological changes significantly impact mechanotransduction and force transmission through the connective tissue matrix, resulting in non-biotensegral, mechano-metabolic processes leading to fibrosis and densification, coupled with reduced mobility and efficiency (Corr and Hart 2013, Pavan et al. 2014).

In such cases, based on biotensegrity principles, disruption to the connective tissue continuum may manifest as pain or result in injury (such as herniation, ruptured tendon, strained ligament or headache) in a weak myofascial location specific to the individual. This translates practically, for example, by saying that it is possible that an incision in the abdomen could cause subsequent local and distant fascial and connective tissue disruption. Such disruption would result in pain being experienced at some distance away, perhaps in the shoulder, knee, foot or neck (ipsilateral or contralateral). The bodywork therapist, movement practitioner or surgeon must extract a detailed history from the patient in order to paint an accurate picture concerning the true source of pain and injury (Stecco et al. 2014).

Acknowledgment

I wish to pay respect and give thanks to the donors, their families and friends, for their precious gift of body donation for the purpose of cadaveric dissection in medical education. In every aspect of my professional life I do my utmost to ensure that all images used provide a powerful educational learning opportunity for the reader.

References

Corr, T., and Hart, A. (2013). Biomechanics of scar tissue and uninjured skin. *Advances in Wound Care.* 2:37-43.

Fitch, M. T., and Silver, J. (2008). CNS injury, glial scars, and inflammation: inhibitory extracellular matrices and regeneration failure. *Experimental Neurology.* 209:294–301.

Grunwald, M. (2016). *Homo hapticus: Warum wir ohne tastsinn nicht leben können.* Munich, Germany: Droemer.

Huijing, P. A. (2009). Epimuscular force transmission: a historical review and implications for new research. International Society of Biomechanics Muybridge Award Lecture, Taipei, 2007. *Journal of Biomechanics.* 42(1):9–21.

Levin, S. (2018). *Bone is Fascia.* Available at: https://www.researchgate.net/publication/327142198_Bone_is_fascia [accessed 30 December 2018].

Pavan, P. G., Stecco, A., Stern, R., and Stecco, C. (2014). Painful connection: densifications versus fibrosis of fascia. *Current Pain and Headache Reports.* 18:441.

Purslow, P. (2010). Muscle fascia and force transmission. *Journal of Bodywork and Movement Therapies.* 14:411–417.

Sharkey, J. (2017). *The Concise Book of Dry Needling: A Practitioner's Guide to Myofascial Trigger Point Applications.* Berkeley, CA: North Atlantic Books.

Stecco, A., Gagey, B., Belloni, A., Pozzuoli, A., Porzionato, A., Macchi, V., Aldegheri, R., De Caro, R., and Delma, V. (2007). Anatomy of the deep fascia of the upper limb. Second part: study of innervation. *Morphology.* 91: 38–43.

Stecco, A., Meneghini, A., Stern, R., Stecco, C., and Imamura, M. (2014). Ultrasonography in myofascial neck pain: randomized clinical trial for diagnosis and follow-up. *Surgical and Radiological Anatomy.* 36:243–253.

Stillwell, D. L. (1957). Regional variations in the innervation of deep fasciae and aponeuroses. *The Anatomical Record.* 127: 635–653.

Tabibian, N., Swehli, E., Boyd, A., Umbreen, A., and Tabibian, J. H. (2017). Abdominal adhesions: a practical review of an often overlooked entity. *Annals of Medicine and Surgery.* 15:9–13.

Tsay, A., Allen, T. J., Proske, U., and Giummarra, M. J. (2015). Sensing the body in chronic pain: a review of psychophysical studies implicating altered body representation. *Neuroscience and Biobehavioral Reviews.* 52:221–232.

Scar tissue in movement

Joanne Avison

Chapter 7

"An astoundingly wide variety of natural systems, including carbon atoms, water molecules, proteins, viruses, cells, tissues and even humans and other living creatures, are constructed using a common form of architecture known as tensegrity. The term refers to a system that stabilizes itself mechanically because of the way in which tensional and compressive forces are distributed and balanced within the structure."

Donald E. Ingber, The Architecture of Life,
Scientific American (Ingber 1998)

Every living thing exhibits unique properties that reflect all kinds of variety and complexity to express themselves as a form. The numerous components of these complexities are exhibited as variously within a species as there are varieties of species to exhibit them. Within each member of a species, the parts which combine to form and express that member are also examples of living things exhibiting unique properties. Each example incorporates its own dynamic patterns, which define it as living, be they the patterns of colour and chemistry, physical, structural or functional shifts, in the everyday matter of being alive. The biology of living matter is a story of systems within systems that combine all the subjects we can study them under. From geometry to geography, history to histology, engineering to embryology and

morphology to mathematics, we can find evidence of an infinite number of subjects in living functioning complexities, such as the human body.

"...yet when they are combined into some larger functioning unit – such as a cell or a tissue [or a whole organism] – utterly new and unpredictable properties emerge, such as the ability to move, to change shape and to grow."

Donald E. Ingber, The Architecture of Life,
Scientific American (Ingber 1998)

Movement is a signal of life. One of the difficulties in writing about the shape-changing qualities that describe movement in all living forms, in any context of scientific reference, is that the living motion of a self-motivated being is not an intellectual process. In living nature the biological process of movement, or self-motivation as a sign of life, is instinctive at its simplest level. Language, while being the intellectual tool of description, can simultaneously become the restriction. As such, in order to develop the theme of this chapter, considering the impact of scar tissue on movement, particularly from a biotensegrity point of view, images have also been used to provide a visual metaphor which speaks to the wholeness of the living biological system that each of us is, as us (Figure 7.1). They also

Chapter 7

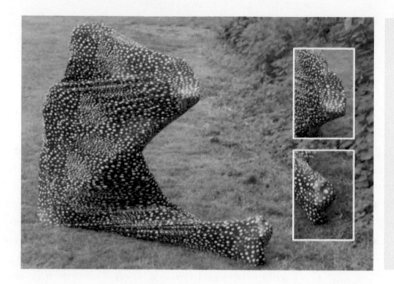

Figure 7.1
This image offers a simple visual metaphor for a pre-tensioned or pre-stressed architecture, presenting the idea that the human body forms in this way, and that all its tissues are animated under conditions of tension-compression, binding forms (and bound forces), united as a whole volume, in the planet's gravitational field.

Image reproduced with kind permission from Art of Contemporary Yoga Ltd. Photographer: Amy Very; model: Helen Eadie; tube provided by Trudy Austin; creative co-ordination: Bex Hawkins.

provide a visual clue as to how forces transmit around wholeness under tension and compression; interrupted by scar tissue, when it too becomes part of the whole. Then, in and of itself, the organism has a new complexity and ever more new and unpredictable properties emerge, along with the new patterns we can learn to incorporate (Figure 7.2).

Working with fascia when scar tissue is involved, movement can become restricted and we are invited to piece together the elements, to gather from all of the chapters in this book some overarching logic which will contribute usefully to whatever individual situations may arise in practice. Looking at this logic through the lens of biotensegrity provides some very useful tenets to encourage manual and movement professionals of all types to consider scars as significant contributors to shape, and therefore also to

movement and postural patterns. We begin and end as volumes in space that express an intimate relationship between the inside forces pushing out and the outside forces pushing in. The membranous interface – be it between the organelle and its surrounding cell, or the organs and their surrounding organismic seal (the skin) – are under tension and compression at all times in all positions at the most basic level of the structure, if biotensegrity is recognized as the founding biological template.

"Biotensegrity is the model that binds."

John Sharkey, Clinical Anatomist
(Sharkey 2015A)

Sharkey (2015A) also suggests that biotensegrity is the "model that binds all other models", a statement which hints at the power of the biotensegrity paradigm, to contextualize the impact of a local insult on the global tissues (also see Chapter 6). Can the scar of having an appendix removed as a teenager affect the ability of the torso to move in multidirectional ways when one is aged 40 to 50 and wanting (for example) to perfect a golf swing?

It is worth considering how biotensegrity assists the overall view, or logic, behind the impact of any scar, on global integrity and structure as well as local glide within the tissue matrix, particularly to the structures in the immediate vicinity of the original scar tissue. It raises questions regarding the overall ability to integrate previously (pre-scar) seamless motion capacity and fluid dynamics, under the new (post-scar) organization. That is, at least from the point of view of morphology and considering the impact on mechanotransduction (Chapter 5), signaling and communication, both at the scar and throughout the body. As we will discover, these aspects can affect movement and motility in all directions, both locally and distally, to a greater or lesser extent.

As its basis, biotensegrity identifies the structural, soft-tissue architecture of a living volume in space that is self-organizing and which defies gravity (Levin 2009). In other words, it can maintain its volume in space to retain its shape and move around without being deformed permanently in doing so. It retains the ability to move itself beyond a

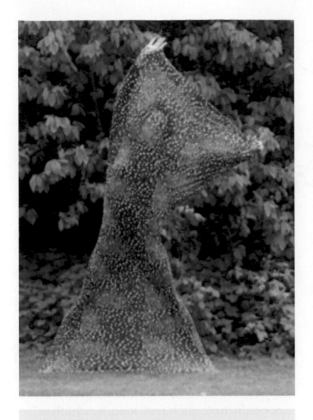

Figure 7.2

As a metaphor for a pre-tensioned architecture, were this net to be cut and stitched back together, it would continue to be under tension, wrapping the compression elements. There would, however, be an inevitable morphological change from such a scar to the tension-compression organization and overall shape of the whole. This would be reflected as a local impact at the site of the repair and, simultaneously, in a different pattern to the overall constraints upon the whole range and scope of motion in making this form.

Image reproduced with kind permission from Art of Contemporary Yoga Ltd. Photographer: Amy Very; model: Helen Eadie; tube provided by Trudy Austin; creative co-ordination: Bex Hawkins.

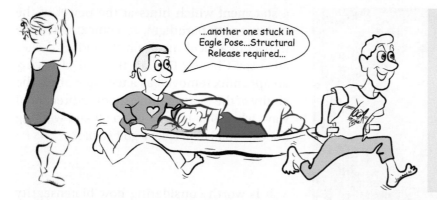

Figure 7.3
Something we are able to take completely for granted is the body's innate ability to restore its shape after changes in movement.

Images: by Joanne Avison; reproduced with kind permission from Art of Contemporary Yoga Ltd.

90-degree angle to the ground while keeping its own innate structural integrity. For example, we do not assume the shape of a chair after we have sat in it, and we also know that once we have reached a complex yoga pose we don't tend to get locked into its form (Figure 7.3). We let it go. In this sense the deformation is temporary and the reformation represents the nature of our ability to readily restore our natural posture, given appropriate time in which to do so. This is known as "innate elasticity" or "energy storage capacity" (Avison 2015B). This global biotensegrity-based pattern, which is also innate to the local tissues (see Chapter 4), is the foundation of our ability to bound, rebound and, as such, bounce back despite insult and injury, to a greater or lesser extent depending upon the specifics of the scar or intensity. The tension-compression relationships may change considerably in the event of insult or injury. However, as Scarr explains (see Chapter 4), we remain organized to evolve with them, to the best of our ability under the circumstances at the time. As living, soft-matter creatures, our architectural design is conceived to reorganize and adapt.

Hard-matter materials, such as those used in the architecture of buildings, in general conform to the rules of static morphologies and stacking. A column, for instance, has to remain at a 90-degree angle to the ground in order to sustain its structural integrity. A tilt in a column supporting a building will severely threaten the entire structural integrity of the hard-matter architecture it supports. However, soft-matter materials do not conform to such restrictions, which raises the question as to why the human or animal spine is referred to in anatomical nomenclature as a vertebral column (Gracovetsky 1985, Levin 1995, Sharkey 2015C) (Figure 7.4).

The classical language restricts us to the terminology of hard-matter physics pertaining to much of our industrial environment. However, definitions for items such as levers, joints, linear bands, flat planes and stacked vertebrae are inappropriate for us as living constructs; these are concepts to which our soft-tissue bodies cannot conform. We routinely bend, twist, fold and fidget into and out of all sorts of shapes and shifts as part of our

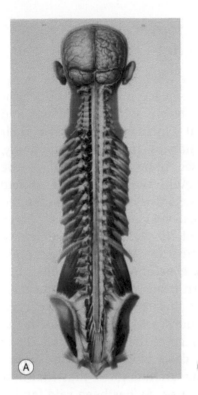
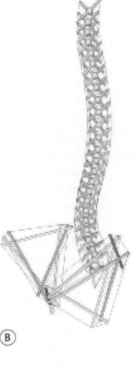

(A)

(B)

Figure 7.4
(A) Vintage classical anatomical image of the vertebral column, which, from a posterior view, presents the spine as if the bones stack to form a column.
(B) A computer-generated design by Tom Flemons (2018), showing a drawing from which he made a tensegrity-based model of the spinal organization. This model makes structural sense of what we can do with the human spine, which functions as many things, but not a column.

Reproduced with kind permission from Art of Contemporary Yoga Ltd.

natural body language, whose mother tongue is gross motion and micro-motility, writ large in the round (Avison 2015A) (Figure 7.5). Our body language is one of curvatures, that is, retaining the ability to restore itself while invariably accumulating a history of adaptation.

The body only attempts to mimic the syntax of rigid, hard-matter mechanisms when specifically trained to appear as though it can; learning to perform robotic dancing is a skill, as is standing still, because both require so much practice. Humans simply don't move like robots and, as such, cannot be readily cut and pasted together, as though the matrix can be fully restored to its original construction by replacing one part with another. Nor can our bodies fully ignore the impact of a cut and its repair; however, they can adapt to many changes in their morphology, as illustrated by the examples given in this book. Robotics and medical advances in designing prostheses can simulate motion, and the ability to replicate movement naturally is being explored in bioengineering research (SunSpiral 2017). Natural living motion occurs in patterns of soft, not hard matter; they are fundamentally distinct and it is important to distinguish between them in order to understand scars and their impact, as viewed from the perspective of biotensegrity.

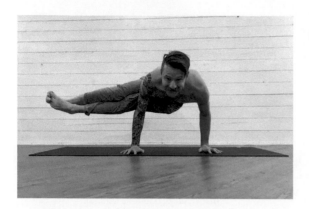

Figure 7.5
If the spine behaved as a column as classically described, it would be impossible to achieve this yoga position – twisted parallel to the ground, supported on the hands.

Model: Wibbs Coulson; www.mandukyayoga.com. Reproduced with kind permission.

Ancient wisdom and new knowledge

In general, our work in all forms of body-work still takes place under the reductionist theories of levers, joints, flat planes and biomechanical explanations that owe their founding principles to classical anatomy, which is based upon the removal of the fascial matrix. With the exception of discrete sections of fascia, this omission has resulted in a gap in the developmental process of how we understand the wholeness observed in every living creature. Whatever the expression or form, everyone we know, love, live with and learn from is whole. Despite their longevity and their popularity, these classical explanations are not expressed in the natural language of the living tissues. They fall short of describing soft-tissue, whole, self-motivating architectures that manifest as living creatures. As has been said (and it bears repeating), the natural language of the living tissues is expressed in continuous and joined up writing in our animated forms, informed constantly by the sensory, communicating nature of connective tissue matrix (Schleip 2003A, 2003B); circulating as (and in) its natural, internal environment, enclosed by its outermost container.

Scar tissue changes the matter of tissues by introducing a new pattern consisting of the entire organization in which it is formed, no matter how small the scar. What is the impact upon the global body of a local scar? And what might be the most valuable logic, or lens, through which to explore it? Treatment is considered elsewhere in the book, specifically referring to the foundation of biotensegrity (see Chapters 4 and 6). When considering the various and valuable assets of this work, how do we make sense of (or extrapolate the logic behind) what actually happens to our movement when there is single or a multiple scar in our structure?

Reductionist classical principles propose that individual muscles are separately attached to bones (at the origin and insertion points), usually working with another muscle (as an antagonistic and agonistic pairing), which causes a joint between two

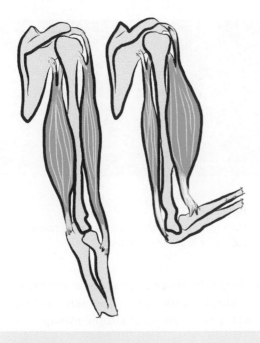

(depending on whether it is a first-, second- or third-class lever and how it interlocks with its neighbors), either joint-by-joint or lever-by-lever. From an engineering perspective there are major issues with this theory (see Chapter 4: closed kinematic chains, pp. 36–40); note also Dr Stephen Levin's famous, crystallizing point, quoted below:

"There are no levers in non-linear biologic forms. Anywhere. Ever."

(Levin 2009)

Also, Jaap van der Wal's vehement comments in personal correspondence to this author:

"Just because it looks like a lever doesn't mean it is a lever".

(Jaap van der Wal, personal correspondence)

Figure 7.6
The classical iconic image of the elbow as a lever; notably, all the neighboring muscles, bones and connections, as well as the connective tissues, have been removed, to itemize and isolate this typical view. Therefore the musculo-skeletal aspect of the whole system is reduced to the locomotive function (and vice versa). The wholeness of the organization is ignored and the continuity of levers from shoulder to fingertips is assumed as a standardized mechanism throughout. By definition, this fact undermines the term lever in its entire application to living bodies and soft matter.

The difficulty is that we have inherited an idea of leverage (as if it is the singular fact applicable to living tissue providing an explanation of skeletal bending moments), which actually applies exclusively to non-living, linear forms that operate under different rules to those determined by hard-matter physics (Figure 7.6). Humans, animals, fauna and flora, insects and even microscopic viruses occupy space as self-assembling entities. They fill (and are filled by) soft matter. Each has different organizational properties that

bones to bend in a certain way as a consequence of one muscle contracting while the other relaxes. This commonly held belief assiduously assigns specific actions to each muscle (via their activating nerves) and to the various structural conditions of each joint give rise to different sets of structural rules. These rules change how scar tissue behavior is explained and treated; it transforms those ideas that suggest it has no impact on movement or, for example, that a scar on one foot can have no effect whatsoever upon the opposite shoulder. From the perspective of biotensegrity, everything affects everything else (to varying degrees) by virtue of a living system's wholeness. Whether that is a detrimental impact, or one which can be overcome and managed by the individual dealing with it, is a distinct and invariably individual matter.

The foundation upon which scar tissue is understood can be highlighted here (along with all the other chapters in this book) and observed in a useful manner, given the visual metaphors which are provided. In an age that understands networks, biotensegrity invites us into the world of soft-matter systems. These are interwoven interdependently and interconnected throughout our form and the forms within it (including those which form smaller networks within the larger ones). Everything is bound together from the outside skin fabric to the innermost bone marrow core by connective tissues, remaining under tension and compression all the time. This means that rather than moving as liquid blobs or rigid robots, we are in a co-ordinated, whole-matter, closed kinematic chain matrix. It is one that can dance along a spectrum of suitable compliance, flexibility and stiffness, which we can change. When we see images of Jean-Claude Guimberteau's endoscopic view of the interior architecture (Figure 7.7)

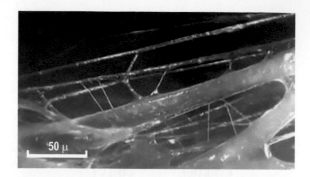

50 μ

Figure 7.7
From *Interior Architectures*, Jean-Claude Guimberteau, 2009–2019 (Guimberteau 2019).

we begin to appreciate a whole new world of complexity underneath the skin. It helps to observe through some simple metaphors.

"As Guimberteau and Delage (2012), Huijing and Baan (2001), and van der Wal (2009), have shown, boundaries in the body are artificial, arbitrary, descriptive conveniences. Tissues in the body are not contiguous, just sharing borders, but continuous, transmuting into one another. The body is an open-office plan, a union of organs united under one roof."

Stephen Levin, *Bone is Fascia* (Levin 2018)

We are bound together as a whole in close-packed variations that resemble the contained froth on a morning cappuccino, more so than they match the lever-arm system of a crane or the workings of a clock mechanism; those principles we inherited from our forefathers in the Renaissance (Avison 2015A). In other words, each and every one of us consists of one piece of bio-origami, organic fabric. This fabric, which is variously and universally called fascia, wraps the innerness of us, every part of it, in all its different kinds of location-specific soup, in multiple folds of that one contained and containing material or body fabric (Sharkey 2015B). It has very specific patterns within that wholeness; nevertheless, its continuity is relentless. The membrane of a disc (*annulus fibrosus*) wrapping its core (*nucleus pulposus*) is quite distinct from the anterior/posterior longitudinal, ligamentous wrapping within which all discs reside. This "ligamentous tubing" forms the sheath that encases all the discs and vertebrae as one continuous spinal structure, close-packed in various biotensegrally organized directions to give us our range of motion, and the ability to hold our spines parallel to the ground without our heads falling off (see Figures 7.5 and 7.8), which they would if the spine formed a column according to the engineering definition of a column. As we know, and can see from Figures 7.5 and 7.8, clearly this doesn't happen.

When the fascial fabric, or body building material, self-assembles, it does so under various conditions and one structural (or architectural) order. There are genetic codes and kinetic impulses that invite it to follow both original and unique patterns. That is according to our species and the specific combinations of the parent genes, and the circumstances and histories of our individual occurrence in the space/time continuum. Whatever those are, nevertheless we begin as one whole complete zygote, wrapped in the *zona pellucida*. This wrapping (meaning transparent membrane)

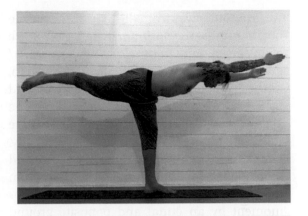

Figure 7.8

In this pose, Wibbs is holding his spine and one leg parallel to the ground. His entire bodyweight is balanced on the small muscles and bones of one foot, none of which are individually capable of supporting that weight at this angle, if the rules of hard-matter architecture were to be applied here. However, closed kinematic chains (see Chapter 4, pages 36-40) explain how Wibbs moves into and out of this posture, as well as holding it in relative stillness, while he breathes and balances.

Model: Wibbs Coulson; www.mandukyayoga.com. Reproduced with kind permission.

folds and enfolds us as part of the continuity in which (and from which) we self-assemble. We do not go into hospital for limb bolt-on procedures (Avison 2015C) to provide future leverage and to equip the embryonic structures to move as such. We form ourselves in motion, as biomotionally whole structures that relentlessly self-assemble as volumes, responding constantly to the forces of our environment at the time. As elemental and subtle as these forces of nature may be, they grow us from the compression (outside in) as we grow ourselves from the tensioning (inside out) to express the optimum balance of nature at any given point in time, as a whole tension/compression volume. In-utero and ex-utero, nothing is added that isn't grown with us (and by us) as part of the process leading from one zygote to one adult. The growing patterns are independent of gravity and yet, paradoxically, once we are born they develop in balance and in response to its demands, matched from movement-to-movement and moment-to-moment by an equal and opposite ground reaction force.

We do not begin life as a flat-packed robot that has to be assembled and moved by outside forces, despite the fact that we birth into multiple external forces which our internal forces have to transmit and translate. Fascia, as a force transmission system, at the very least has to calibrate these forces universally throughout the system and invariably distribute these forces economically, via the path of least resistance (see Chapters 4 and 5 for more detail). As a model that binds and distributes forces heterarchically as well as hierarchically, biotensegrity provides an explanation for the economy of speed and spread of this force transmission throughout all non-linear, biologic forms. The body doesn't get to bend only at the knee or elbow. Even before the limbs have formed, while they are growing out of their preceding buds, they communicate and respond, within and without, to these forces of genetics, kinetics and containment. They are built of the fabric that is growing them, into which they grow, invariably under tension due to differing growth rates and the emergent properties of every differentiation; repeating the quotation that opened this chapter:

"An astoundingly wide variety of natural systems, including carbon atoms, water molecules, proteins, viruses, cells, tissues and even humans and other living creatures, are constructed using a common form of architecture known as tensegrity. The term refers to a system that stabilizes itself mechanically because of the way in which tensional and compressive forces are distributed and balanced within the structure."

Donald E. Ingber, The Architecture of Life,
Scientific American (Ingber 1998)

Despite the species-specific pattern that generated their ideal morphological properties, any whole living structure is engaged in this global organization of the local allocation/differentiation of where and when to organize the forces it transmits. They are invariably distributed throughout the entire system, using various miracles of diffusion, transmission, signaling, communication, distribution and mechano-transduction. This brings about the balancing of forces and forms at the most incredible levels of detail and complexity, to manifest the metamorphosis we are all destined to experience. As Jean-Claude Guimberteau wrote in the narrative to *Interior Architectures* (Guimberteau 2019), "Why question a daily miracle?" An answer to that question may be that we need to understand the basis of how continuous the process of deformation and reformation is to the living tissues on every scale – and biotensegrity explains this. Therefore, we can begin to understand some of the issues and complexities of scar tissue when it is imposed upon the original system(s) and its innate weave or patterns (Snelson 2010).

At the gross level of organization, the bony arrangements tension the softer

---

Box 7.1 Case study

As a hand surgeon, Dr Guimberteau (Guimberteau 2019) has produced stunning video footage of living tissue under the skin. On one occasion he described exquisitely detailed surgeries in which, through extreme skill, patience and microsurgery (and a profound understanding of fascia and its many characteristics as a pre-stressed architecture), he restored movement after debilitating injury. It is worth referring to one particular case as we emphasize the adaptive nature of the living tissues, rather than suggest that scars are innately negative.

Guimberteau described one case of a man with a badly injured forearm (after an accident), which, despite the bony tissue mend, was left almost immobile and certainly unable to flex. In this case, the patient's own latissimus dorsi muscle was used to graft and transplant new tissue where it had been destroyed, bringing undamaged myofascial material and neurovascular vessels to a new site, where they had to learn

to behave differently as flexors of the forearm (somewhat divorced from their usual neighbors at the posterior thoracic tissues and humeral head!). It was clear that Guimberteau, his colleagues and the patient agreed that, given the accident, it was worth the sacrifice (and more scar tissue) to reintroduce motion to the forearm and learn to move with less "myofascia" on the latissimus dorsi donor site.

In France, morning coffee is an essential ingredient to one's peace of mind. This custom is mentioned here, because through appropriate motion and more than 12 months of careful rehabilitation, the result was extraordinary. "We had to first ensure the fascia and myofascia were integrating...then to allow the various neurovascular vessels to work within the transplant site and reorganize appropriately, in their own respective timeframes." Guimberteau explained that: "The nerves took much longer... however, they were eventually reintroduced to their new role and our friend can enjoy picking up his cup and drinking his morning coffee."

Guimberteau was at pains to explain the issues and advantages of transplanting and slowly introducing the patient's own tissues, to restore motion to the forearm, wrist and hand, which took a long time, but was worth the sacrifice given the extensive damage to upper limb and hand mobility. The injury rendered the forearm immobile and the rehabilitation was long and not always easy. However, by relying upon the adaptive nature of the body to bring about a new expression of morphology, the prioritizing of limb function over the role of the latissimus dorsi muscle brought about a profound improvement for this patient.

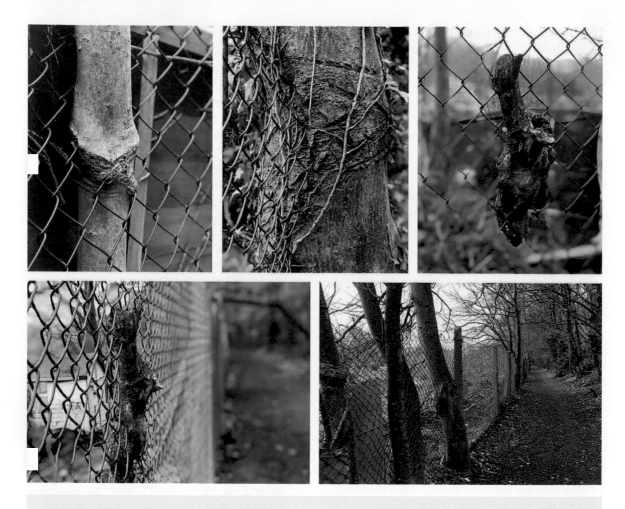

Figure 7.9

This tree has grown around and through the fencing; its agency to grow includes the scars imposed by the fencing material, designed as it is like a closed kinematic chain, albeit man-made. The lattice allows the tree to grow and move with the prevailing winds as the tree does not prevent the barrier from moving and supporting the boundary it marks. Note the top right image which shows where the scar became so strong that the tree surgeons had to cut the branch away from it.

Image by Joanne Avison; creative co-ordination: Bex Hawkins.

tissues and the softer tissues compress the bony arrangements, so they work mutually. So too, the outside forces of gravity compress the body and the inside forces of ground reaction force tension the body so that we can stand up and move around in all directions. Actually, we are (like all vertebrates and viruses) expressing our nature as auxetic materials that abide by very different rules to those governing concrete or even more organic materials, such as pine tables and chairs hand-made with curves; these are man-made wooden structures. We are much more like the naturally self-assembled living trees themselves in their original living form. We are a lot more mobile but operate under the same architectural rules that govern all bound living forms. We manage our priority of mobility in an internally enclosed and more fluid (mobile) medium than that of the tree's interior architecture. Trees manage their stability in an internally more stable medium, binding their roots to the earth. Between us, we share the spectrum of opposite ends of the scale in many ways, breathing in the gases trees release and breathing out those that they absorb. These symbiotic relationships are profound. Nature uses common assembly patterns for all of us, we just speak her miracles in different morphological dialects. Nevertheless, all abide by the soft-matter rules of each species' specific articulation, literally and symbolically (Ingber, 1998, 2008).

Biotensegrity provides the grammar, vocabulary and syntax that describes those rules and invites us to realize that scar tissue in a tree is much like scar tissue in a body; it affects our forming process and changes our movement patterns, just as it changes the shape of a tree and its growth pattern.

In Figure 7.9, the natural growth pattern of the tree could be said to have evolved to manage the restrictions offered by the fence and continue with its purpose to grow into the woodland where it resides and co-hosts the forest floor (Wohlleben 2017) as part of this forest community. If the definition of evolution is to "include and transcend that which precedes" (Wilber 2001), then we might say that the tree has evolved to manage the scar tissue and grow itself appropriately, given that restriction and its nature to optimize force transmission and adapt accordingly, via the path of least resistance.

Scars

In the human body, consisting as it does of one complete fabric, folded and enfolded in many different twists, turns, pockets and places, scars paradoxically repair and cut continuity, simultaneously. They may look like thin lines on the skin, however, in the human dissection laboratory, particularly in soft-fix Thiel dissection (Sharkey 2015A) (see also Chapter 6, where this is thoroughly investigated), it is apparent that the body responds naturally and vigorously in some cases, to what might be described as the repair process, post-injury or post-insult. For example, behind a thin, 10 cm-long line in the skin (depending upon location), it has been witnessed that there may be several centimeters of thickening along the length and width of the scar, underneath the skin, through the superficial and deeper fascia. There can also be ribbon-like structures extending beyond the site, as if to anchor to other neighboring structures or to form some kind of stability (see Figure 6.1).

This process of how fascial tissues respond to scars has invited more research in recent years, including work by Bove and Chapelle (2012) demonstrating that scar tissue formation is a natural response that can be affected and possibly ameliorated with appropriate touch. Given the component of time (e.g., considering how long after the scars were formed that treatment took place), this light touch can be unreasonably valuable (see Chapter 5). Similar to the tissue transplant case (Box 7.1), quoting Dr Ida P. Rolf, it clearly takes "the compound essence of time" to change the information being signaled through the tissues, where that may be possible or advantageous. Perhaps it can be considered, as a result of Bove and Chapelle's (2012) research and others, that the right palpatory application, at an appropriate depth, speed, rate and frequency, can change the emergency state of repair to one more akin to the original order?

The answer to that question is explored elsewhere in this book and forms the basis of the clinical experience behind the treatments discussed. However, the point which should be emphasized, is that the body (however zealously) is not necessarily fighting itself when a particular scar tissue restricts motion. Initially at least, it is compelling to consider that the body is seeking to mend itself and limit the damage, even if the binding mechanism and material triggered in order to achieve that is occasionally more than is actually required. In other words, because we are living, biological forms, the tissue matrix receives the signals that the cut, wound, surgical incision or insult have changed the

status quo and damaged the wholeness or integrity of something somewhere in the joined-up matrix of the body's volume. The body appears to seek, just as it originally self-assembled, to self-repair. Essentially, by mobilizing various natural wound-healing procedures, it does exactly what we would do if we found a hole or tear in a woven shopping bag we were carrying: we would tie a knot in the net. As simplistic as that may sound, it is what we effectively see in the tree (Figure 7.9) and is what actually happens in the body, as evidenced in soft-fix cadaveric dissection (Sharkey 2015A) (see also Chapter 6).

A knot in the net, an example to visualize

At the simplest level, imagine a patterned stocking (similar to the ones illustrated in Figures 7.1 and 7.2) with a cut or tear through the fabric. By wrapping a contained volume, this cut has two clear areas of morphological impact, among many more subtle ones. First, the compromised integrity of the cover, or wrapping, is affecting the volumetric nature of the function of covering – meaning, it cannot do what it is designed to do, which is to seal or protect or distinguish or differentiate that which it covers and interfaces. The tensional nature of the stocking, along with its wrapping function, has effectively lost its original integrity, or wholeness, thus it leaks and exposes that which it wraps.

Second, from what might be compared to a more histological point of view, the actual tissue/fabric has lost its integral or local weave pattern, and so it can no longer shape-shift with the movements of that which it wraps in the same way. It won't glide so easily within and around that which encases it, or which is enclosed by it. Note that this impact also includes that which the wrapping encloses.

To put it bluntly, the fabric is not fit for purpose unless its wholeness can be restored (i.e., suitably bound), as well as other properties listed for consideration (see later). Were this to be a waterproof covering, for instance, it now allows in water; were this to be any form of membrane protecting what is inside it from what is outside it, then that protection has been compromised by the damage to the membrane or interface. If we stick with this metaphor and picture something as simple as a hole in a sock, we may find ourselves walking along irritated by the lack of the protection the sock now affords the heel, and/or the nature of the hole that now wraps our big toe if that is where the sock was damaged or the hole first appeared.

We might then darn the sock (i.e., knot the net) to repair the damage and bind the hole, which would be similar to the effect of wound-healing mechanisms in the body. Here is where the metaphor can help to invite the sense and logic of what happens in the body regarding movement. Metaphorically, reading "darn = scar" and "sock = original fascial tissues" (and weave thereof), there are many microscopic and macroscopic details that will be affected, which include but are not limited to:

- The darn tends to have different qualities/weave to the rest of the fabric.

- The area around the darn, where it may be thickened, may be vulnerable to that difference.

- The "felt sense" of the fabric or weave of the sock is less compliant at or around the darn.

- The density of the fabric is palpably changed.

- The frictionless gliding of the fabric interfaces between the structures may be compromised.

- The effect on the elasticity of the whole sock is marked.

- The movement potential within the sock is different.

- The overall shape of the sock has changed.

- As a material that also filters things through it, that woven architecture (filter) is compromised.

- As a material that transmits forces along it, that tensional equilibrium will have changed.

- As a material that transmits forces around it, that surrounding organization will have changed.

- As an enclosing membrane, the containing morphology and function will have changed.

- As a tensioned web, essentially, that tissue resonance will have changed.

Even when using an example as simple as a sock, it is relatively easy to imagine that without it the shoe rubs on the skin, the skin produces a blister and friction results in injury to the living tissue (or the neighboring material). There are essentially no layers in the human body (Sharkey 2015A), they are artifacts of dissection, revealed by the process of cutting (the word "anatomy" comes from the Latin meaning "to cut up"). However, there are clear distinctions between different types of fabric and certain qualities that are distinguished by the same fascial tissue that connects them. (Welcome to the paradoxical world of fascia!) We have not started to consider the specific tissues that may have been cut and the consequential global impact. Suffice to say that there are multiple aspects to be considered and it is the function on many levels (both global and local) that inevitably has to adapt to the change in structure. In a sense, nothing is unaffected at the most subtle level.

From the perspective of the fascial matrix as the largest sensory organ of our form (Grunwald 2008, Schleip 2003A, 2003B), rather than experiencing these limitations and changes in the quality of the sock material by touching it, in the case of a living scar we are the material or fabric being described and we sense (and suffer) those changes from within and around the damage to the tissues. The metaphorical knot in the net may be saving the primary function of sealing the system, however, such increased density of the fabric will inevitably involve neurovascular vessels, muscle tissue, fascial expressions of tendinous or ligamentous discontinuity and any

aponeurotic sheaths that may have been cut through. The fluids moving through them, as well as the forces they foster and modify, will also be interrupted, resulting in the need for new patterns and morphologies to be adopted and adapted to. Surgeries and injuries involving visceral operations have to cut through such tissues and body walls before reaching the organs or tissues they seek to repair. Any broken bones, whether or not they require plates or pins, will also retain bony scars in this, the hardest in the spectrum of fascial soft tissues (Levin 2018) (see also Chapters 9 and 10 for scar treatment approaches).

Force transmission (Figures 7.10–7.13)

Movement is the keystone theme within the biotensegrity paradigm; any movement expresses mechanical forces through the system distributed via the most efficient route, be they low or high threshold, gross or micro-motilities within vessels. Thus any block in force transmission (Langevin et al. 2011), such as that which a scar could create anywhere, will apply to overall motion as well as to fluid dynamics within the local tissue at the site of injury. A difficulty in using the sock metaphor is that the sock is not entirely continuous: it only encircles the foot! It stops being a sock at the ankle or the knee, depending on its length. By adopting the same rules that levers don't work (there are no open two-bar chains in the body), then socks don't work either (they have an end). A sock doesn't stop being a sock.

As obvious as "We don't stop being a sock" sounds, it does appear to be an issue for people

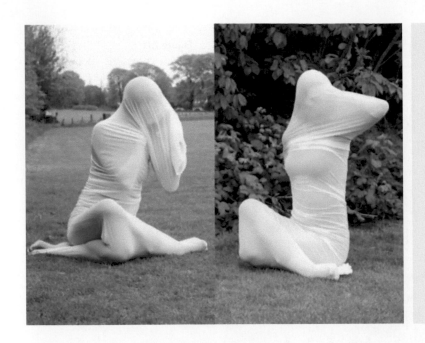

Figure 7.10

In these images, whatever movements Helen performs inside this tubing (which is not entirely enclosing, but is close) reveal the different shapes she is making through the folds and bands that move with her, changing as she moves. It is a visual metaphor that indicates the forces being continuously transmitted through the fabric wrapping her, inside which she is acting as a compression provider to the tensioned "skin" of the material.

Image reproduced with kind permission from Art of Contemporary Yoga Ltd. Photographer: Amy Very; model: Helen Eadie; tube made by Stephani Neville; creative co-ordination: Bex Hawkins.

learning about biotensegrity. Your outer "skin sock" is not only continuous around the perimeter of your body volume, but it also continues along the inside. From mouth to anus, as per your pre-embryonic forming architecture, you were formed out of one fabric. It may have a very squiggly, multiple-folding inner tube, but your body form is essentially one long toroidal pattern, woven together in multidirectional wholeness, to and from one original piece as a self-containing volume. Cut it and it seeks to self-assemble a suture, "stitching" itself together or reinforcing the tissues to fortify the break in continuity. In dissection it can be seen that the binding of scar tissue can also appear to be anchoring the "stitches and the weave" to other neighboring vessels or forms, to strengthen and fortify the cut and possibly modify its impact. Scar tissue may be one of your fascial net resources, performing its naturally responsive

damage-limitation technique, regardless of the reason for cutting. It may be very valuable and life-saving, such as the surgical removal of a foreign body that was life-threatening, or as in the case of Guimberteau's patient (Box 7.1) with the restored ability to flex his forearm. However, the act of "darning the [continuous] sock" has an effect upon the continuity, the suppleness, the mobility and weave of the fabric, and its organizational relationships to that which it surrounds, echoing throughout the entire organism. A more useful symbolism may be to consider a scar as a "seam in the structure", because many of the reasons for scarring are relatively valuable, especially when it comes to life-saving surgeries and recoveries. Even in cuts and grazes, the body is predisposed to heal itself and tie the knot! Figure 7.13 shows movements and the shadows of their transmission vectors within a tensioned tube.

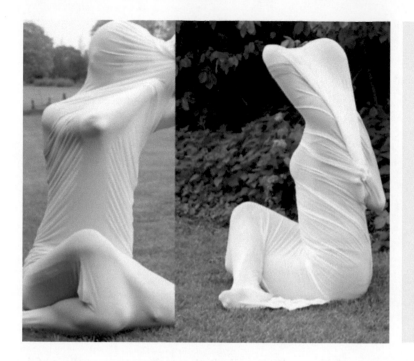

Figure 7.11
In these images, the shadows in the fabric indicate that the pull or force vectors, or folds, wrap around the volume continuously.

Image reproduced with kind permission from Art of Contemporary Yoga Ltd. Photographer: Amy Very; model: Helen Eadie; tube made by Stephani Neville; creative co-ordination: Bex Hawkins.

However we acquire scars (and most of us do), they have an impact on movement to a greater or lesser extent. We might conclude, therefore, that it is worth having appropriate scar tissue treatment to counter the possible impact of scars and to restore optimum movement to tissues, given appropriate timing, frequency and rate of change, and the limitations or reasons for the scar. It is also interesting to note that similar adaptation techniques in manual therapy can be gently accumulated to restore motion where scarring can sometimes restrict it. It is interesting to speculate whether the research cited in this chapter (Bove and Chapelle 2012) regarding gentle massage, might apply to gentle movement. Is it possible that subtle, small movements (or micro-movements) may indeed serve scar tissue in a similar way towards the gradual and cumulative results of gentle palpation from a practitioner? This would be with a view to rehydration, reorganization and re-establishment of integrity or, at the very least, moving towards it. On a spectrum of gentle to strong, appropriate movement (i.e., from micro-movements to macro-movements) at low frequency, accumulating towards higher frequency over a sufficient time period for the individual situation, would provide adequate re-adaptation time, to the extent that the weave could be restored in the direction of its optimal pattern. In all cases, it could be proposed that, just as light touch from without works, so might light motion from within. If it can have a suitable body-wide impact (however small the movements may seem to be), then like all medicine, it will be a matter of dose and degree for that individual, to embody the value of such gentle rehabilitation. As in the

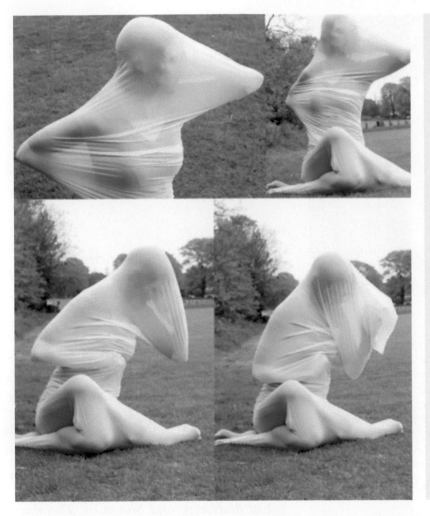

Figure 7.12
In these examples, the bands in the fabric represent the forces being transmitted through it, which are continuous in their pattern around Helen.

Image reproduced with kind permission from Art of Contemporary Yoga Ltd. Photographer: Amy Very; model: Helen Eadie; tube made by Stephani Neville; creative co-ordination: Bex Hawkins.

case of Guimberteau's client (see Box 7.1), it was a year before forearm flexion could be achieved – a year of subtle, slowly accumulated adaptations to the overall tissues.

At the very least, this global explanation of impact relates to the local injury, and local treatment can clearly affect the global comfort and motion patterns (see the case studies in Chapter 11). However individual the cases may be, it is a lens worth looking through when considering scar tissue in motion. In the instance of the visual metaphor (Figure 7.13), a seam in the structure may be essential to the overall integrity of the organism, given the insult or injury. That is, whether we like it or not, a scar may be a repair and on the basis of survival, a great alternative. The scar represents inevitable changes in force transmission;

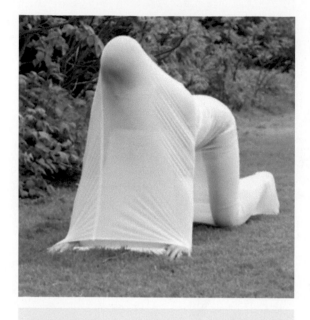

Figure 7.13

The material shows, through the light and shadows playing over this visual metaphor, how forces appear to continuously wrap around whatever is tensioning them – except when there is a seam. They are still transmitted; however, it is possible to see here how their surrounding pattern is interrupted, whatever that may mean in an individual situation and the living tissues it affects.

Image reproduced with kind permission from Art of Contemporary Yoga Ltd. Photographer: Amy Very; model: Helen Eadie; tube made by Stephani Neville; creative co-ordination: Bex Hawkins.

the invisible nature of tension and compression that we can't immediately see but which biotensegrity accommodates and explains so beautifully. It describes the nature of our self-assembled metamorphosis and resilience as we continue to grow through life, scars and all. The fascial matrix is ubiquitous, so when any scar forms it affects the entire organization

to varying degrees. The biological tensional integrity (or biotensegrity) requires that it must "self-bind" to restore that integrity. That is what nature designs it to do.

"Biotensegrity is the model that binds – and it binds all the other models."

(Sharkey 2015A)

References

Avison, J. S. (2015A). The Science of Body Architecture. In *Yoga: Fascia, Anatomy and Movement,* pp. 33–53 (1st edition). Edinburgh, UK: Handspring.

Avison, J. S. (2015B). *Yoga: Fascia, Anatomy and Movement,* pp. 137–158 (1st edition). Edinburgh, UK: Handspring.

Avison, J. S. (2015C). *Yoga: Fascia, Anatomy and Movement*, pp. 74–99 (1st edition). Edinburgh, UK: Handspring.

Bove, G. M., and Chappelle, S. L. (2012). Visceral mobilization can lyse and prevent peritoneal adhesions in rat model. *Journal of Bodywork and Movement Therapies.* 16:76–82.

Flemons, T. (2018). intensiondesigns.ca. Available at: http://intensiondesigns.ca [accessed 17 September 2019].

Gracovetsky, S. (1985). An hypothesis for the role of the spine in human locomotion: a challenge to current thinking. *Journal of Biomedical Engineering.* 7:205–216.

Grunwald, M. (2008). *Human Haptic Perception: Basics and Applications.* Basel, Boston, Berlin: Birkhäuser.

Guimberteau, J.-C. (2019). endovivo.com. Available at: http://www.endovivo.com/fr/architectures,interieur,dvd.php [accessed 17 September 2019].

Ingber, D. E. (1998). The Architecture of Life. *Scientific American.* 278:48–57.

Ingber, D. E. (2008). Tensegrity and mechanotransduction. *Journal of Bodywork and Movement Therapies.* 12:198–200.

Langevin, H. M. (2011). Fibroblast cytoskeletal remodeling contributes to connective tissue tension. *Journal of Cell Physiology.* 226:1166–1175.

Levin, S. M. (2009). Biotensegrity.com. Available at: http://www.biotensegrity.com/resources/tensegrity--the-new-biomechanics.pdf [accessed 18 September 2019].

Levin, S. (2018). *Bone is Fascia.* Available at: https://www.researchgate.net/publication/327142198_Bone_is_fascia [accessed 17 September 2019].

Levin, S. M. (1995). *The Importance of Soft Tissues for Structural Support of the Body.* Philadelphia, PA: Hanley and Belfus.

Schleip, R. (2003A). Fascial plasticity - a new neurobological explanation: Part 1. *Journal of Bodywork and Movement Therapies.* 7:11–19.

Schleip, R. (2003B). Fascial plasiticity - a new neurobioligcal explanation: Part 2. *Journal of Bodywork and Movement Therapies.* 2:104–116.

Sharkey, J. (2015A). Dundee University Soft Fix Dissection Programme (NTC). Interview, 29 June 2015.

Sharkey, J. (2015B). One Series: One Net. Interview, October 2015.

Sharkey, J. (2015C). Terra Rosa eMagazine, issue 16. Available at: https://issuu.com/terrarosa/docs/terra_rosa_emag_issue_16 [accessed 11 February 2020].

Snelson, K. (2010). tensegritywiki.com. Available at: https://tensegritywiki.com/wiki/Weaving#Links_and_References [accessed 17 September 2019].

SunSpiral, V. (2017). magicalrobot.org. Available at: http://www.magicalrobot.org/BeingHuman/2017/01/my-2016-nasa-ames-summer-series-presentation-superball-a-biologically-inspired-robot-for-planetary-exploration [accessed 17 September 2019].

Wilber, K. (2001). *A Theory of Everything.* Boston, MA: Shambhala Publications.

Wohlleben, P. (2017). *The Secret Life of Trees* (paperback edition). London, UK: William Collins.

Emotional aspects of scars

Jan Trewartha

Contribution from Katerina Steventon

Chapter 8

Scars and somatic memory

Once we are able to work effectively with scars, it is easy to just focus on the scar itself because we cannot wait to get started, knowing the difference we can make. But there is no such thing as a scar without the person behind it. An understanding of the effect of a scar on someone is vital; we need to work with the whole person, taking into account any fears, anxieties, trauma or body image issues they may have, as well as the history of the scar and the events which surrounded its creation.

Therapists are used to their clients' emotions surfacing during treatment, for example, grief and anger, and these are taken as a healthy sign of letting go of any feelings the client has been holding on to. Often this happens in the days after treatment, when the client might report crying for a day or more or having dreams in which unresolved issues appear to be addressed by their subconscious.

Memories can also surface and, when working on scars, clients may recall the process of being anesthetized or the sadness they felt at losing control during the birthing process when their planned natural birth became an emergency cesarean section (C-section).

Recollections of the fear or pain of surgery or injury may also pour out of them, and they can be left with a feeling of relief, bringing grateful tears or laughter.

These experiences are common, and lead us to the literature in search of answers; some of the myriad and varied comments and research on this topic follow below.

Walt Fritz (2018) warns that: "For too long the occurrence of emotional feelings/responses during a manual therapy engagement have been twisted to be seen as a statement and belief that emotions are somehow stored with [sic] the tissues being treated. While touch is powerful and helpful, caution needs to be taken not to confuse safe therapeutic touch allowing an emotional response...with stories of how fascia/muscle/etc. are the vessel of those emotions." There is, clearly, a difference between the two responses, but what scientific support is there for somatic memory?

Van der Kolk (1994) states: "Ever since people's responses to overwhelming experiences have been systematically explored, researchers have noted that a trauma is stored in somatic memory and expressed as changes in the biological stress response. Intense emotions at the time of the trauma initiate the long-term conditional responses to reminders of the event, which are associated both with chronic alterations in the physiological stress response and with the amnesias and hypermnesias characteristic of posttraumatic stress disorder (PTSD)."

Tozzi (2014) explores many possible ways in which the fascia may hold memories, from the irritation of primary afferent nociceptive fibers to the effect of substance P on the collagen structure: "into a specific hexagonal shape, referred (to) as 'emotional scar'", and from epigenetics to a: "'body consciousness' functionally interconnected with the 'brain consciousness' of the nervous system, via the crystalline liquid medium of the ground substance." He concludes that: "...it is suggested that a possibility may exist that manual therapy might affect various forms of memory, producing profound tissue changes from subatomic to global effects."

Myers (2014) responds to Tozzi's article but prefers not to use the concept of tissue memory: "My own experience is that 'memory', whatever it is, manifests as a distributed phenomenon across all the body systems – perhaps in the shape and resonance of the fascial 'liquid crystal', but also emotionally written in the chemistry of the blood, lymph, peptides, and transmitters, and obviously in the patterned firing of the nervous system." Preferring to ask whether fascia contributes to awareness, rather than memories, Myers continues: "Again simply on the basis of my experience, I find that the fascial system holds the form of memory or consciousness that we commonly call our belief systems. I do not mean belief systems like '-isms' – capitalism, communism, or any religion – but the underlying beliefs about ourselves that get 'written' into our form through trauma or repeated actions or postures. I change my ideas through changes in neural firing. I change my feelings through changes in fluid chemistry, but I change my fundamental 'stance', or attitude...Through a change in the patterning of the fascial net...the fascial net developed in concert with the neural net and the circulatory net, and has never been separate, so they all act in concert." Could, therefore, a restriction in the fascial net caused by scarring, where structures become adhered together and fluid flow can be affected, change how we feel about ourselves and alter our attitudes?

Rothschild (2000, p. 45) discusses the phenomenon of flashbacks that: "involve highly disturbing replays of implicit sensory memories of traumatic events". The sensations that accompany them are so intense that the suffering individual is unable to distinguish the current reality from the past. A flashback: "... can be triggered through either or both exteroceptive and interoceptive systems. It might be something seen, heard, tasted, or smelled that serves as the reminder and sets the flashback in motion. It can just as easily be a sensation arising from inside the body. Sensory messages from muscles and connective tissue that remember a particular position, action, or intention can be the source of a trigger." This is known as state-dependent memory. Thus, it is feasible that a surgical experience could resurface when lying supine and receiving therapeutic touch, or that the therapist's hands on the scar might stimulate traumatic recall.

It would seem that the jury is still out on this fascinating topic, but research continues.

Our reactions to scars

Apart from those more subtle ways in which traumatic injury or surgery can affect us, the actuality of the physical scar can also take its toll.

Relationships are the hidden casualties of some scars (e.g., C-section scars, episiotomies that have gone wrong). When a woman cannot bear to look at or touch her own scar (a very common occurrence), she may well not be able to allow a partner to touch it, disliking that part of her body so much that sexual intimacy is affected. Some women report feeling a failure after a C-section, due to their inability to have given birth normally, or feeling "less of a woman" after a hysterectomy or mastectomy, with an irretrievable loss of their sense of femininity. Fear, loss of control and anger are all emotions that can be held around the scarring and may affect how a woman feels about herself. Later in this chapter we

will look at how people can develop a positive attitude towards their scars, learning to accept them as part of who they are, and as landmarks on their life's journey.

With the more visible scars, Western society can be more accepting of a scarred man than of a scarred woman. A man's facial scar might imply that he has fought and is therefore "tough". Face and body scars can become badges of honor; a deep cut on the cheek from a descending garage door might transform, in the telling, into a tale of defending someone when young. Al "Scarface" Capone is a legendary case in point; Capone would usually claim that his scars were war wounds, rather than resulting from a bar fight when a smaller man slashed Capone's face for insulting his sister (Capone 2018). Interestingly, it is difficult to find a photograph of Capone with his scar; the majority have been taken at an angle so that the scar is hidden.

Some scars are beyond such concealment. Our faces are our interface with the world; through them we express our emotions. We communicate, see, speak, laugh and cry. Damage to the face disrupts that medium because facial scarring can leave the face less supple and therefore less communicative. Our sight and speech may also be affected, depending on the extent of the devastation wreaked by, for example, an injury, tumor or burn. Acid burn scars, with their resultant tissue destruction, are equally life-altering. "Every year, an estimated 1,000 women are attacked with acid in India. However, there is little official data on these assaults; most cases go unreported and unregistered." Acid attacks are often intended to disfigure women who refuse to marry a man or deny their sexual advances. They have also happened amid family conflicts, domestic violence and spousal abuse. Usually premeditated, and aimed at the victim's face, the goal is long-term damage (Mahendru 2017).

The Katie Piper Foundation is well known in the UK, founded by former model Piper (Figure 8.1) following an acid attack in 2008 that led to multiple operations. The foundation offers immediate care for burns victims, from leaving hospital to rehabilitation, medical tattooing for lost eyebrows and lips, hair transplants and replacements. The foundation's vision is: "to have a world where scars do not limit a person's function, social inclusion or sense of wellbeing" (Katie Piper Foundation 2018). By using her public profile to raise awareness, Piper has empowered herself and given hope to others.

In India, the Sheroes Hangout café in Uttar Pradesh aims to restore confidence to women with severe facial burns after acid attacks (Figures 8.2–8.4). The social inclusion referred to in the Katie Piper Foundation's vision statement is challenged when the visible damage causes a reaction from others of horror and avoidance, but Sheroes provides a haven, work and acceptance; they lead the way, showing the world that it is time everyone is accepted for who they are

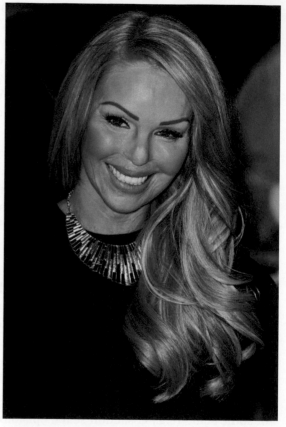

Figure 8.1
Katie Piper.

Photo credit: Shutterstock.

and that scarring does not change the inner person.

These attempts to leave someone with life-long, visible scarring are deliberately designed to efface a person. "Mohammad Jawad, a plastic surgeon who helped rebuild Katie Piper's face and works with victims in South Asia, says

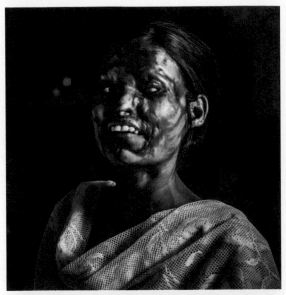

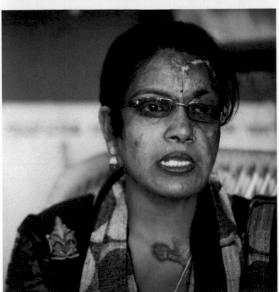

Figures 8.2 and 8.3
Sheroes provides support and helps restore confidence.

Photo credit: Hashim Ahmad Hakeem.

the crime is about trying to destroy someone's identity" (Castella 2013). Even the words we use clearly express what such scarring is considered to do to someone: deface ("to destroy or mar the face or external appearance of, to disfigure: to obliterate") and disfigure ("to spoil the figure of: to change to a worse form: to spoil the beauty of: to deform") (Schwarz et al. 1990). It must take huge courage, support and an ability to stand up and be who you are to overcome such a devastating blow to one's sense of self, and it is heartening that our society's attitudes are changing, while surgical techniques, medical tattoos, skin camouflage and other support systems are enabling people to retake control of their lives.

The possible results of disliking our scar

Feeling antipathy towards our scar may well affect our body image and self-worth, as well as our ability to be intimate with another person. But does it affect us on a deeper level as well? Sharkey (Chapter 6) points out that: "Interoception can modulate the exteroceptive representation of the body, while setting parameters concerning pain tolerance. Structural changes in the connective tissues, such as scarring, fibrosis and adhesions may dysregulate the pathways that are responsible for providing details concerning the status of one's structural state and could therefore cause a distortion of our own body image."

Lipton (2018) discusses telomeres, the noncoding extensions at the end of DNA. When

DNA self-replicates, the strand length reduces a little each time. At first, the telomeres act as a buffer zone that protects the genes at the ends of the chromosomes, and for a long time it was believed that this reduction in length was the ultimate cause of aging and disease, and thus determined how long a person could live. However, in 1978, Blackburn and Gall discovered that the enzyme telomerase adds length to the telomeres, thus allowing for continuous cell division without losing the coding part of DNA.

What stimulates telomerase? Lipton goes on to suggest that epigenetic factors – good nutrition, exercise, a positive outlook, self-love, being loved, being useful/needed, a sense of security and a "Bring it on!" attitude to life – all do this. On the other hand, poor nutrition, childhood abuse, domestic violence, PTSD, chronic stress, having no purpose in life, and being isolated and unloved all reduce telomerase production. However, someone under chronic stress who nevertheless deals with it positively rather than feeling victimized, will still have good telomerase production. Cellular longevity is affected by our state of mind, continues Lipton, and not having any purpose in life can be read as "I don't have any reason to be here"; this, he suggests, is why so many people die shortly after retiring as they feel less useful, and that feeling inhibits telomerase production.

Lipton (2008) cites Pert (1999), whose "elegant experiments established that the 'mind' was not focused in the head but was distributed via signal molecules to the whole body." Also, that "through self-consciousness, the mind can use the brain to *generate* 'molecules of emotion' and override the system. While proper use of consciousness can

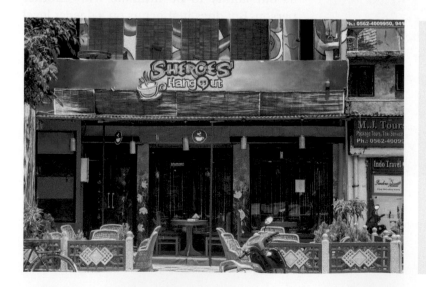

Figure 8.4
The colourful Sheroes Hangout exudes a feeling of welcome.

Photo credit: Hashim Ahmad Hakeem.

bring health to an ailing body, inappropriate unconscious control of emotions can easily make a healthy body diseased."

Learning to love ourselves

Shame, anger, hatred, low self-esteem, embarrassment and depression: these are just a few of the powerful emotions that can be generated by scars. Our scars can affect the clothes we wear (for example, wearing trousers covering a scar on our legs if we dislike showing it), the makeup we feel we need to hide them, and how we perceive ourselves. Time can bring acceptance, as can receiving scar therapy or using commercial products designed to optimize the scar.

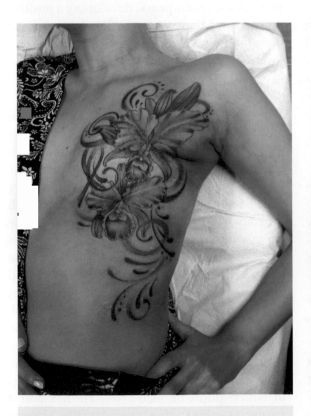

Figure 8.5
Breast tattoos can help a woman take back control of her body.

Photograph reproduced by kind permission of Gilded Lily Design, paramedical body art clinic.

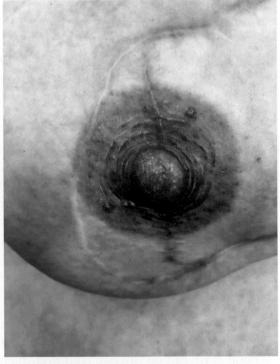

Figure 8.6
A tattooed nipple can restore symmetry and a feeling of completeness.

Photograph reproduced by kind permission of Yorkshire Mastectomy Tattoos.

Generating a positive attitude to our scarring will help our physical health as well as our self-image. Making something beautiful from a scar is one way of doing this and tattoos are an increasingly popular choice as people re-empower themselves. As one woman, post-mastectomy, who decided to have the area tattooed, put it: "I'm more body-confident now than I have ever been. I feel as if I've taken control not only of my body, but of myself as a woman. I've taken a life-changing and potentially detrimental experience and turned it into a real positive" (Fletcher 2018). Note that this kind of tattooing (Figure 8.5) is a specific skill and uses high quality, permanent inks; therefore, the artist must be professionally trained.

Post-plastic surgery reconstruction, the nipple, so potent in its symbolism of womanhood and motherhood, can be skilfully tattooed to look three-dimensional, restoring symmetry and a feeling of completeness (Figure 8.6).

Children and their scars

How do we teach a child to love or at least appreciate their scar when they are bullied at school? If we can do this, we empower them. We could say, for example, how important the scar is because it stands for something that has changed their lives, be it a cleft palate repair, or recovery from an accident or injury. By understanding the difference the operation, and thus the scar, has made, the child can often feel positive towards it, perhaps even grateful, and thus find it easier to stand up to bullies at school. The scar can become a badge of honor and a source of pride, symbolic of a challenge which has been overcome. Parents can also, as appropriate, encourage a variety of exercises to help maintain a good range of movement and full joint and soft tissue mobility, including running, jumping, skipping and dancing. Hobbies that inspire children and get them out playing with their peers, developing a positive attitude and body image, will help. If the scar does not make a child unhappy then the bullies have no weakness to pick on.

Bullying will always be a challenge for children who stand out. "Kids are pretty much guided missiles when it comes to finding every bump, every scar, every nose made out of an old toe that they can find, and they did" (Hoge 2015). Robert Hoge was born with a tumor from the top of his forehead to the tip of where his nose should have been. His eyes were pushed to the side of his head "like a fish". His mother rejected him at birth until she was persuaded by his siblings to accept him and bring him home from hospital. Robert had multiple operations, including the creation of his nose from one of his deformed toes, until at the age of 14 he was given the choice of whether to have further surgery, at which point he said "No". He has had a career as a journalist, speechwriter, science communicator for the Commonwealth Scientific and Industrial Research Organisation and a political advisor to the former Queensland Premier and Deputy Premier, and has "owned" his face: "It's the choices that matter. My ugliness made it easier for me to own my face than many of you." "Choose to own your face. Understand all the love, all the life and all the pain that is the art of your face." Hoge chose the path of owning who he is.

The traumatic effects of child circumcision

Procedures such as circumcision in male babies, and female genital mutilation (FGM) in girls up to the age of 15 (illegal in the UK), are both often performed without general anesthetics, although male circumcision in hospital employs anesthetic creams. These are the most intimate form of assault, whatever the reason may be. Research into male circumcision has associated it with severe pain, "increased irritability, varying sleep patterns and changes in infant-maternal interaction", changes to developing neural pathways and other responses (Goldman 1999).

"Research has demonstrated [that] the hormone cortisol, which is associated with stress and pain, spikes during circumcision... Although some people believe that babies 'won't remember' the pain, we now know that the body 'remembers', as evidenced by studies which demonstrate that circumcised infants are more sensitive to pain later in life" (Narvaez 2015). "Women who have undergone FGM are more likely than those without FGM to experience painful intercourse, reduced sexual satisfaction and reduced sexual desire ...FGM may lead to sexual phobia... Women may also experience more difficulty reaching orgasm, and shame or embarrassment about

intimacy... Narrowing of the vaginal opening may make intercourse painful for both partners" (Chung 2016).

Society's attitudes to scars

From tribal cultures to gang cultures, scarification or cicatrization (the deliberate creating of patterns, words or identifiers on the body) is used to confirm the individual's place as a member of a group. At the other end of the scale, self-harmers can be equally ritualistic in the branding, scarring or burning of their skin. "Repressing intense emotions for extended periods of time can lead to emotional numbness. Immediately following a trauma, a temporary repression of emotions can be functional, but long-term this coping strategy can be costly. After conditioning oneself not to feel, it can become difficult to reawaken one's emotions. Many young people who have coped by repressing feelings eventually have difficulty feeling anything. So, to feel, they cut. One reason teens may turn to physical pain as a coping strategy is that they are terrified of emotional pain, feeling that it might overwhelm them; as a result, they seek out physical pain so that they can feel something, but something much less threatening than emotional pain. Others who self-harm do not repress their emotions. Instead, they experience the full intensity of painful emotions but have difficulty managing them. They may self-harm in order to redirect their attention from those emotions to a more manageable, controllable type of pain. This redirection allows them to temporarily disconnect from the emotional pain and achieve a sense of relief and mastery" (Davenport 2016).

Box 8.1 Scarring and the epidermal barrier (envelope)
Katerina Steventon

The skin consists of three distinct layers, the epidermis, dermis and hypodermis. The skin as a whole, but in particular its very top layer, the stratum corneum layer of the epidermis, forms a barrier protecting our body. It creates a boundary, dividing our insides from the outside world, preventing water loss, bacterial ingress and sunlight-induced inflammation. Research shows that the skin can sense external information such as sounds, scent and light, in the same way as the brain (Denda and Katsuhiko 2017). The skin is our largest sensory organ and an emotional envelope, reflecting the emotions felt by our body by changes of their parameters in color, for example: we blush when embarrassed or turn pale when frightened. The integrity of the layer is essential; epidermal keratinocytes are tightly adhered to each other by cellular junctions. The dermis is rich in extracellular matrix, and especially collagen, and provides the majority of the tensile strength of the skin.

In case of an injury, when the skin is cut, burnt or abraded, the body makes a desperate attempt to close the skin fast at the expense of a quality repair, resulting in scar tissue. Even minor damage to the skin, such as the removal of cells in the upper layer of the epidermis, initiates a cascade of immune-mediated events, involved in repairing the skin barrier immediately after the injury.

Newly formed scar tissue has a stratum corneum that is dysfunctional. Its inadequate barrier leads to dramatic increases in water loss, skin dryness and changes in the biomechanical functioning (Rawlings et al. 2012). Barrier function is reduced in scars compared with healthy skin and only improves with scar maturation (Gardien et al. 2016). Scars have an increased number of fibroblasts with a change in fibroblast phenotype and collagen orientation (Moortgat et al. 2016). Keloid and hypertrophic scars, resulting from the overproduction of collagen by fibroblasts during wound healing, are associated with changes of intrinsic cellular mechanical properties. It is stiffness of the skin tissue that determines the regenerative ability during wound healing (Hsu et al. 2018).

Dehydrated scars are often pruritic and painful due to the impaired epidermal structure. The reduced number of sebaceous and sweat glands causes a lack of the reservoir of stem cells and hydration. The epidermis of a scar is thinner and vulnerable; the dermis has abnormal orientation of collagen matrix, impacting negatively on the barrier function. An impaired and incompletely re-epithelialized epidermis is deficient in protective features and reacts more sensitively to external factors. It is also susceptible to penetration and bacterial infections leading to inflammation (Busch et al. 2018). Skin hydration controls the epidermal expression of specific cytokines and growth factors. The effects of the swelling impact the signaling (through stretching or compression) as keratinocytes are connected to each other. Hydration improves softness and smoothness of the skin, and restoration of barrier function controls the scar formation; studies conducted in vitro using keratinocytes and fibroblasts showed the direct effects of hydration, suppressing collagen production in fibroblasts thereby reducing excessive scarring. Hydration regulates epidermal cytokine production increasing the ratio of anti-fibrotic/fibrotic cytokines to reduce hypertrophic scar formation (Tandara et al. 2007).

Epidermal barrier recovery is delayed by psychological stress (e.g., academic exams or divorce). The hypothesis of the epidermis, the

continued

interface between the body and the environment, as a "third brain" seems viable as it has many of the functional activities of the brain. Epidermal keratinocytes express a variety of environmental sensors (temperature, mechanical stress, chemical stimuli) and secrete a range of hormones and neurotransmitters that influence the whole-body state and emotions. In laboratory culture, keratinocytes can generate electrochemical patterns similar to those of the brain and express all the components of the stress-related hypothalamo–pituitary–adrenal (HPA) axis (Denda 2015).

The paucity of keratinocytes and an inadequate barrier in a scar make it less able to sense and respond to the external environment or reflect the internal state of the body. This creates an environment that is barren, stiff and mute, lacking in communication. Gentle touch may impact the mechano-transduction pathways to release the tension associated with scar retraction and induce apoptosis of myofibroblasts, leading to softening and integration of the scarring within the body in both the physiological and psychological sense.

Whatever its history, any scar can be owned so that it becomes a symbol of pride or of overcoming adversity. The perception of our scars by our families, our societies and our friends, as well as our concept of what constitutes beauty or good looks, may influence our acceptance, or otherwise, of our scar. However, just as society is dropping its rigid evaluation of people by their disability, skin colour, gender, appearance or mental state, so scars will become more and more part of someone's identity and history and not something to be judged.

References

Al "Scarface" Capone. (2018). Available at: https://en.wikipedia.org/wiki/Al_Capone [accessed 28 December 2018].

Blackburn, E., and Gall, J. G. (1978). Available at: https://en.wikipedia.org/wiki/Telomere, reference 11 [accessed 9 September 2019].

Busch, K. H., Aliu, A., Walezko, N., and Aust, M. (2018). Medical needling: effect on moisture and transepidermal water loss of mature hypertrophic burn scars. *Cureus.* 10:e2365.

Castella, T. (2013). BBC News Magazine. How many acid attacks are there? Available at: https://www.bbc.co.uk/news/magazine-23631395 [accessed 28 December 2018).

Chung, S. (2016). 28 Too Many. The psychological effects of female genital mutilation. Available at: https://www.28toomany.org/blog/the-psychological-effects-of-female-genital-mutilation-research-blog-by-serene-chung/ [accessed 30 December 2018].

Davenport, J. (2016). Sunrise Residential Treatment Centre. The truth about cutting and self-harm. Available at: https://www.sunrisertc.com/truth-about-cutting-and-self-harm [accessed 29 December 2018].

Denda, M. (2015). Epidermis as the "Third Brain"? *Dermatologica Sinica.* 33:70–73.

Denda, M., and Katsuhiko, S. (2017). Skin is the Mirror of the Heart. Available at: https://www.shiseidogroup.com/advertising/talk/7.html [accessed 15 December 2018].

Fletcher, G. (2018). The Impossible Body: Instead of a scar I had a piece of art: women on their post-mastectomy tattoos.

Available at: https://www.theguardian.com/lifeandstyle/2018/sep/22/instead-scar-piece-art-women-mastectomy-tattoos [accessed 28 December 2018].

Fritz, W. (2018). Where does somatic memory in the body reside. Available at: http://www.fascialfitness.net.au/articles/where-does-somatic-memory-in-the-body-reside/ [accessed 10 August 2019].

Gardien, K. L., Baas, D. C., de Vet, H. C., and Middelkoop, E. (2016). Transepidermal water loss measured with the Tewameter TM300 in burn scars. *Burns*. 42:1455–1462.

Goldman, R. (1999). The psychological impact of circumcision. *BJU International*. 83 (Suppl. 1):93–102.

Hoge, R. (2015). Ted Talk. Own your face. Available at: https://www.youtube.com/watch?v=QbxinUJcLGg [accessed 27 November 2018].

Hsu, C. K., Lin, H. H., Harn, H. I., Tang, M. J., and Yang, C. C. (2018). Mechanical forces in skin disorders. *Journal of Dermatological Science*. 90:232–240.

Katie Piper Foundation (2018). Available at: https://katiepiperfoundation.org.uk/ [accessed 28 December 2018].

Lipton, B. (2018). The Healing Power of Gratitude - Bruce Lipton Explains Telomeres. Available at: https://www.youtube.com/watch?v=vEfXK3D8vGc [accessed 29 December 2018].

Lipton, B. (2008). *The Biology of Belief*, page 102. London, UK: Hay House.

Mahendru, R. (2017). 50.50 gender, sexuality and open justice. Available at: https://www.opendemocracy.net/5050/ritu-mahendru/india-cafe-sheroes-fights-back-acid-attacks [accessed 28 December 2018].

Moortgat, P., Anthonissen, M., Meirte, J., Van Daele, U., and Maertens, K. (2016). The physical and physiological effects of vacuum massage on the different skin layers: a current status of the literature. *Burns & Trauma*. 4:34.

Myers, T. (2014). Myers' response to Tozzi's editorial. *Journal of Bodywork & Movement Therapies*. 18:599–601.

Narvaez, D. F. (2015). Psychology Today. Circumcision's psychological damage. Available at: https://www.psychologytoday.com/gb/blog/moral-landscapes/201501/circumcision-s-psychological-damage [accessed 30 December 2018].

Pert, C. (1999). *The Molecules of Emotion*. Pocket Books. UK: Simon & Schuster.

Rawlings, A. V., Bielfeldt, S., and Lombard, K. J. (2012). A review of the effects of moisturizers on the appearance of scars and striae. *International Journal of Cosmetics Science*. 34:519–524.

Rothschild, B. (2000). *The Body Remembers*. New York, NY: W. W. Norton & Company.

Schwarz, C., Davidson, G., Seaton, A., and Tebbit, V. (1990). *Chambers English Dictionary*. Edinburgh and New York: W & R Chambers.

Tandara, A., Kloeters, O., Mogford, E. J., and Mustoe, T. (2007). Hydrated keratinocytes reduce collagen synthesis by fibroblasts via paracrine mechanisms. *Wound Repair and Regeneration*. 15:497–504.

Tozzi, P. (2014). Does fascia hold memories? *Journal of Bodywork & Movement Therapies*. 18:259–265.

van der Kolk, B. A. (1994). The body keeps the score: memory and the evolving psychobiology of posttraumatic stress. *Harvard Review of Psychiatry*. 1:253–265.

A different approach to working with scars

Sharon Wheeler

Contribution from Wojciech Cackowski

Introduction

Sharon Wheeler is a Structural Integration practitioner who originally trained with Dr Ida P. Rolf, the founder of Rolfing. Sharon started developing ScarWork more than 45 years ago and it is her own, original work. So far there has been little research, yet Scar-Work is being taught and practiced worldwide due to its tangible results. Here, Sharon discusses her own approach to scars.

The beginning

ScarWork emerged from my Structural Integration practice in 1973. It shares some general philosophy and basic orientation with Structural Integration, however, the hands-on working techniques for ScarWork are completely different. ScarWork seems to affect only the scar tissue and not much else. Working with scar tissue is like speaking a different language in the world of fascia.

I was in the process of giving Joan (not her real name) a standard Structural Integration 10 session series. She had been in a car accident 15 years earlier. The car's steering mechanism failed. With no control, she veered across the oncoming lanes, just missing a head-on collision with a semi-truck, and tumbled down the embankment on the far side. She was not wearing a seatbelt and was thrown halfway out of her window. As the car rolled, both of her legs were broken. Her left leg did all right, but her right leg needed surgery.

Her surgeons operated five times through the fascia lata. They even shaved off part of the head of the fibula before they gave up and told her that she had better keep what she had because if they kept going, she may well end up worse. Her right knee was unable to bend to 90 degrees. It was difficult and painful for her to walk or sit for any length of time. She managed her long-term problems with muscle relaxants and pain medication "every day by noon". Joan was also a nurse and she helped me understand what had happened to her medically.

Her scar was about 16 cm long. Thickened, vertical edges formed a square hollow with a gap so deep and wide I could hide my finger in it; 3 cm either side of the incision were stiff, shiny, irregular ripples with random blotches of red and white coloration. Large areas were still numb.

Dr Rolf had advised me to ignore the scar and establish the function, but this strategy was not working for Joan. One of the major functional goals of the third session of

Structural Integration is to free the knee so that it can move straight forward and back. I was not having any success. In truth, I was having a fair amount of trouble in establishing any kind of knee movement at all. This impressive scar with its adhesions seemed to be the problem. I wondered if something good might happen if I could soften up the scar a little. I had no idea what to do so I allowed my hands to work by feel. I took what I knew about changing tissue from the perspective of Structural Integration and applied it to the scar on a micro-level.

Joan was quite comfortable with what I was doing, so we started a conversation about the movies showing at the town's cinema. We discovered that we shared an appreciation for the wit and talent of Marilyn Monroe.

For about 20 minutes I worked on the bottom half of the scar. When I stopped to see if I was making any progress, I was surprised to see that the square gap was gone, the edges were together, and the ripples on the sides of the scar were smooth and supple. Joan reported good sensory nerve function. The color of the scar matched the rest of her. The surface of the skin had normal polyhedral lines with a matte finish and what looked like fine fuzzy hair.

I asked Joan to sit up and take a look at her scar. She looked it over, touching and feeling it, then said, "I didn't know you could do that." I replied, "Me neither."

When I started to work again, I realized that I did not remember a single thing that I had done.

So I restarted our conversation about Marilyn and the movies, and did my best to let my fingers fly, hoping I would find my way back to what I had been doing previously. Somehow this strategy succeeded. As I worked, I took a little peek now and again. I was able to match up the top half with the bottom half and know what I had done. It felt like normal tissue. Neither of us could find any irregularities left in the texture of the scar. With the scar out of the way, I found the fibula and got it unstuck. This allowed Joan's knee to bend most of the way and she could walk and sit without pain. Joan was able to stop taking all of her medications. Her scar has stayed good to this day. I hope Joan is pleased to be remembered as the beginning of ScarWork. I incorrectly assumed that I had figured out what everyone else already knew. I saw a sign advertizing massage on scar tissue in Carmel, and I remember wishing that I had taken that class. I gave myself a small, congratulatory pat on the back for finding out how to work on scars all by myself and carried on without saying much about it to anyone.

My clients allowed me to explore their scars and I became fascinated. This was very different work from the depth and power of Structural Integration, which I dearly love. The profound results of this light, easy, happy and painless work are a mystery to me.

Eventually, the word got out that I did "things that worked for scars". Some of my colleagues asked for advice so I published an article called "On Scar Tissue" (Wheeler 2008). I was hoping to exchange information with my colleagues. I did not get any new information back, but I did receive requests to run classes. I reframed my publication as a ScarWork manual and designed a workshop format to reflect the spirit of the work. Teaching pushed me to develop ways to communicate the content. I had to unpack the elements of each of the different techniques for my students and identify and clarify some basic principles. I started teaching with 12 techniques; today there are over 30. Periodically, I edit the Scar-Work manual to reflect ongoing growth and development.

Each class I teach is a flood tide of new experiences and information. I get to work on all of the students and all of the class models who volunteer from the local community for free work on their scars. Classes are a total immersion in the subject of scars, and this leads to innovation. For me, classes are like Christmas!

Preliminary research

Communicating with medical people requires science and science requires numbers. Medical imaging can provide some acceptable measurements to generate the numbers necessary for science. I am fortunate to have encountered some excellent researchers. It looks like we will shortly have the opportunity to start a scientific inquiry.

I have some preliminary research to share, consisting of a set of three ultrasound images, which were presented at the Fascia Research Congress in Washington DC in 2015 (Wheeler et al. 2015).

Kristi Blessitt, MD, a gynecological surgeon, took the images and interpreted them. My colleague, Richard Ennis, B.S., did the scientific writing, and I did the Scar-Work. A Mindray DC-6 Doppler Ultrasound machine (2.5-6.0 MHz) was used for all of the imaging. Images were taken before and after a single, one-hour long session of ScarWork.

Subject number 1

The first subject was a 66-year-old woman with a single 43-year-old midline abdominal scar. She had been in a car accident and the front of her body had impacted on the steering wheel. She was losing blood pressure and her doctors performed emergency exploratory surgery, repairing several sites of internal bleeding. She still experienced pain and could feel a strong pull from her scar, especially when she stretched her hands above her head. After ScarWork, her abdomen was smooth and soft. She was pain-free with no pulling (Figures 9.1A & B).

- 'Before' ultrasound taken:
  6 January 2012

- ScarWork treatment given:
  21 January 2012

- 'After' ultrasound taken:
  26 February 2012

Before
Skin to scar: 1.79 cm

After
Skin to scar: 2.74 cm

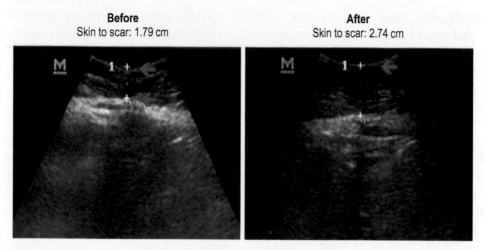

A 0.95 cm increase skin to scar after ScarWork

Figure 9.1A
Before and after ultrasound images for Subject number 1.

Before
Fascial "bleb" at closure

After
Fascial "bleb" is integrated

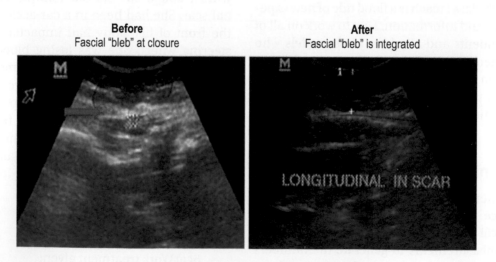

Restoration of normal fascial layers of tension to abdomen

Figure 9.1B
Before and after longitudinal view ultrasound images for Subject number 1.

Subject number 2

The second subject was a 58-year-old woman with three surgeries: a 22-year-old ileo-anal anastomosis, a second ileo-anal anastomosis of 20 years, and a 15-year-old cesarean section (C-section) (see Figure 9.2).

- 'Before' ultrasound taken: 1 July 2012
- ScarWork treatment given: 16 July 2012
- 'After' ultrasound taken: 3 August 2012

Before
Skin to scar: < 1 cm

After
Skin to scar: 2.25 cm

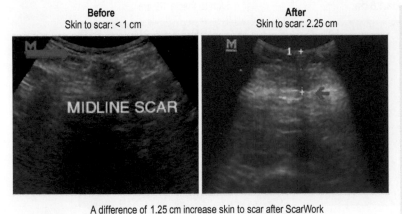

Figure 9.2
Before and after left lateral ultrasound images for Subject number 2.

A difference of 1.25 cm increase skin to scar after ScarWork
Restoration of normal fascial layers of tension to abdomen

Subject number 3

The third subject had undergone three abdominal surgeries: a 30-year-old left sided tubal pregnancy that had ruptured, a 27-year-old C-section, and a 12-year-old hysterectomy (see Figure 9.3).

- 'Before' ultrasound taken: 1 July 2012
- ScarWork treatment given: 16 July 2012
- 'After' ultrasound taken: 3 August 2012

Before
Tubal pregnancy scar at arrow

After
Tubal pregnancy scar released

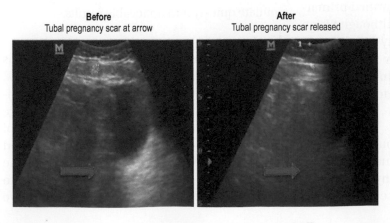

Figure 9.3
Before and after tubal pregnancy ultrasound images for Subject number 3.

Subject Number 3: Control

Dr Blessitt wanted to see what ScarWork would do to normal tissue. After ScarWork, the skin to scar distance only increased by 0.1 cm.

This number was not sufficiently large to be considered statistically significant, which suggests that ScarWork does not affect normal tissue (Figure 9.4).

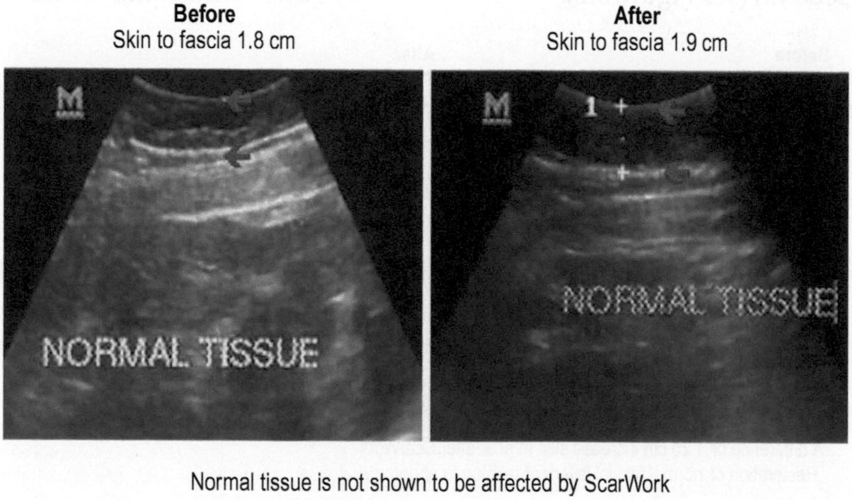

Before
Skin to fascia 1.8 cm

After
Skin to fascia 1.9 cm

Normal tissue is not shown to be affected by ScarWork

Figure 9.4
Before and after control ultrasound images of normal tissue for Subject number 3.

ScarWork orientation

ScarWork is a tactile art form. The goal is smooth tissue. The work is performed primarily through the sense of touch, although vision does play a part. I only use my hands to do the work. I do my best to follow the tensional vectors by feel as my hands seem to sense and know the most about tactile matters.

I work with the intention of putting the scar back together, reversing the damage, mending the tissue, and reassembling any misaligned, surgically created layers. I counter every tensional vector in the fascia head on, directly, with just enough pressure to free a tiny bit of scar tissue. These small, nearly undetectable changes accumulate quickly into noticeable results.

I have observed most impaired functions re-establish themselves with ScarWork. These improvements are fortuitous, unintended, and a source of great delight. They are so common that I use them as indicators of how well a session is going. I have noticed that these functions return during the time of the session and then continue to improve markedly over time. Sensory nerve function and sometimes motor nerve function returns. Internal organs function better. Lymphatic and blood circulation improve. Tissue strength and flexibility improve.

The individual techniques do not reliably produce one particular functional result. The return of impaired functions appears as a by-product of smoothing the whole scar. When the scar tissue feels like normal tissue it starts to function like normal tissue. Possibly the form of the tissue has something to do with its function?

I have respect and a high regard for scars. They consist of precisely the right stuff needed for remediation. They are a treasure trove composed of good tissue that is stuck together all "cattywampus", to use one of Dr Rolf's favorite words.

Every single scar is unique. Cross typing and matching scars and techniques looking for shortcuts does not work as well as hoped. An appendix or C-section scar does not always receive the same techniques or the same sequence of techniques.

Natural scars from an accident or injury are all one of a kind. There are so many variables in a fall down the stairs or a car accident that it is easy to understand each natural scar being different from any other.

Surgical scars are also one of a kind. The way a surgical procedure is performed depends on who the surgeon studied with, at which hospital, and during which years.

Another source of variation in scars is the healing. An infection may alter the surgeon's good work and produce many more adhesions. Stitches may tear out, metal plates and pins are put in and taken out, and a surgical procedure may require several revisions. Scars can get complicated.

ScarWork can be used with people of any age. Because it is painless, even babies usually tolerate it with a smile. Some of my colleagues have used ScarWork with animals and have reported success.

It does not appear to matter how old a scar is. Mature scars of many years are easy to work on with excellent resolution. ScarWork seems to work for most scars. To date, keloids are the one exception, although we are starting to develop techniques that appear to help.

The scar is not merely a mark on the skin, it is connected from the surface of the skin down into the farthest reaches the surgeon explored, including the fluid pools. While the surgeons are in there to remove an appendix, they may decide to take a look at the gallbladder. The scar develops fascial adhesions to all of these places. The entire scar is an irregular, three-dimensional form with odd asymmetric appendages.

Keyhole or laparoscopic procedures are popular for many kinds of surgeries. Patients like them because of the small surface scars. However, if you include all of the tunnels the surgeon makes from the surface incisions to the area of interest, then the amount of scarring is more extensive than a single incision directly over the area. The tunnels are not easy to find. The leakage of fluid from the severed tissues blurs the outline of the tunnel, making it feel amorphous. If you tug on the little surface scars, you will feel the tunnels. Use your other hand to feel for the connection and locate their direction.

Scars feel different from the surrounding, undamaged, normal tissue. The texture is uneven. The textural quality may consist of lumps, holes and strings with stiff, dense areas. These elements have tensional vectors. I work to counter head-on each tensional vector with just enough pressure to win. The scar resolves in the reverse of the direction that created it. Using precision in countering these tensional vectors increases the speed and quantity of change. I experiment with pressure, using different angles, shear, rotation and velocity until I find something that changes the scar, and then I use repetition. When the change rate slows down, I look for a more productive way through the tissue.

I take on what is the most obvious in the moment. I go to the worst, most dense places first as those are the easiest to find, and they will yield the most good. I cannot plan strategies and protocols in advance.

ScarWork is a continuous tactile exploration into the unknown, similar to exploratory surgery in medicine. If I can get the scar tissue unstuck it "goes home". In my experience, and as demonstrated by the ultrasound scans shown above, it does not end up randomly adhering to some other place where it does not belong, forming new adhesions and causing more trouble.

If I cause pain by pressing too much or trying to go too fast, the tissue has a way of keeping me out. It feels like the threatened tissue locks arms with its neighbors and won't let me in to help until I mind my manners.

I try to work without causing any pain. I need feedback to avoid causing pain because there is no way to know if there is pain unless people tell you. If there is pain, I try adjusting my touch to be lighter or I change techniques. In hypersensitive situations, I move far away from the painful area to a place where the tissue is not painful and then work my way back towards the painful area. If the hypersensitivity resolves, I can work on the scar.

If a scar is pain-free and comfortable, I can allow my touch to become more casual and flowing. When the work feels really wonderful, I can allow for a bit of enthusiasm – which looks a lot like working with bread dough.

I ask people to test their range of motion, feel the texture of their scar, and give me a report periodically. This informs me, allows them to track their progress, and gives them an opportunity to talk about their experience. Knowing their stories helps me make sense of the tensional vectors.

Starting to work on scars
Cautions and contraindications

Always work within the guidelines of your therapy profession, as defined by the professional body you are registered to in your country. The guidelines below are in addition to your standard considerations for treatment.

- Before you work with a client, make sure they are signed off by their surgeon and are safe for work. This is normally six to eight weeks post-operation.

- We advise not working on inserted mesh. Mesh used in breast reconstruction does not have the problems of abdominal/pelvic mesh and is safe for work.

- For a client with a recent history of cancer, we recommend requesting a letter from their oncologist to confirm the client is safe for work.

- We advise not working on pregnant women.

- The scar should not be open, infected, inflamed, weeping fluids, or very painful. Tenderness is acceptable.

- Do not work if there is redness or swelling around the scar due to radiation therapy.

- Do not use abrasion on keloid or hypertrophic scars.

- Do your best to work without causing your client pain.

Techniques

All of the work is based on countering tensional vectors. Techniques are ways of working that I have identified as having a pattern. If that pattern works for many people, it becomes a technique. Some of the techniques are more general and all-purpose; others are specific for a particular tissue arrangement. The names given to the techniques reflect the playful quality of this work.

Techniques are best learned in a classroom. Teachers help students calibrate the right kind and depth of touch. Watching a video to learn tactile techniques doesn't give you everything, but videos are better than anything else, and we have included five techniques with videos to guide you as you start to explore working with scars. The descriptions which follow are provided for use with the videos. Visit http://wheelerfascialwork.com/library/videos to watch "Five ScarWork Techniques", or scan this QR code:

Feather Light Sweeping

Use Feather Light Sweeping to start work on most scars. It provides an opportunity for an overall exploration of the extended area and it starts to soften the texture of the scar. When in doubt, go lighter.

If you used a long flight feather, it would approximate the proper amount of pressure for sweeping. I use a single finger because it keeps my enthusiasm in check. More fingers can be used depending on the size of the scar and the angles you need to generate. This does much more than you would expect, so do not skip it to get to the other techniques.

My sweeping finger is moving before making contact with the surface and moving as it breaks contact with the surface. There is a slight drag to the motion, much like petting a small mouse. Sweep towards the scar from all around and through the areas where there may have been swelling and bruising. Bracing or stabilizing the tissue with my other hand yields more change at a faster rate. Bracing uses a light, resting, relaxed contact without stretching or pulling.

The sweeping is performed from the bracing hand towards the scar. Go up to the scar but do not cross the midline of the scar. You do not want to pull the scar apart; you want to put it together.

This technique may seem simple but do not underestimate it; giving it plenty of time will improve the resilience of the skin; it appears to work on the free nerve endings under the skin, and will generally improve the look and texture of the area.

The Cat

The Cat is particularly well suited for abdominal scars and adhesions. It is also useful in many other areas. When you are not sure what to do, try The Cat.

Both relaxed hands sink into the tissue, resting the weight of your arms from your shoulders. Your whole hand stays in contact while gently pushing with a fluid rolling wave. This motion resembles the Hawaiian hula dance hand gesture for "ocean".

Alternate your hands and keep moving your contact around as you work. It does look a lot like kneading bread dough, and very much like a cat. It is easy, relaxed and casual. Work from both sides of the body for balance. It should feel wonderful for the client.

Scraping

Use one hand for scraping and one for a brace.

When surgeons make a minimal incision, they must stretch or retract the tissues wide open to create enough room to work in. It feels like some of the tissues get stuck in the retracted position. This leaves wrinkles under the surface. Scraping smooths and flattens wrinkles.

I use the example of making a bed: if you miss pulling a blanket layer flat in the middle of the process, it leaves a wrinkle under the top layer. You can scrape that blanket layer smooth through the top layers rather than undoing everything to make the blankets lie flat and smooth.

Partially curl your fingers and slowly and gently scrape through the tissue from the brace to towards the scar. Pick up your fingers and do this again in the same direction. Go up to the edge of the incision but not over the edge or down the center of an incision.

Matching Layers

Matching Layers is a complex technique that has several elements to be considered.

Adapt your hands to the constraints of the location, size and shape of the scar. Use both hands.

For longer scars, make contact with the whole hand, using a flat contact. Your hands are a mirror image of each other with your index fingers parallel and one finger on each side of the scar. Drop both hands down

slightly to capture the two large sheets of tissue that form the two sides of the scar. We refer to sheets and layers as artifacts created by surgery or damage.

Start working away from the edges of the scar and push your hands together to push up two rolls of tissue, one on either side of the scar. There is an optimum distance away from each scar and finding it requires a little experimentation. Move the rolls forward and back to the comfortable excursion limit of the skin to address any displacement in the plane that is horizontal to the body surface. Work along the entire scar. Move the rolls up and down to address any displacement in the vertical plane.

Along with the forward and back and up and down motions, tilt each of your hands into different angles or planes. Experiment with some wiggling as you push the two sides towards each other. This motion is similar to pushing two hairbrushes together to interdigitate the bristles.

Down the Rabbit Hole

This technique is used when a scope has been inserted into the body (during laparoscopy or arthroscopy), and also for drain sites or cannula insertions. The scope or drain being inserted and removed creates local trauma and tracking adhesions. With drains, there is simply a straight in and out sensation, but where a surgeon has been investigating, you will feel yourself being pulled into the different areas where that scope has already gone. This technique is based on intention as much as anything else, so keep your focus on your fingertip.

Put your fingertip on the scar. In navel laparoscopy scars this is sometimes impossible, so just put your finger in the navel. Do not apply pressure. Just stay there, very lightly, and follow the tissue; you will usually feel it moving under your finger. If there is anything to clear, you will feel the tissues drawing you in until it might feel as if your finger is fully inside the body. The client may also feel this, as the intention and touch appear to transmit into the deeper fascia. When the movement eventually stops, you will feel as though you are being pushed out; that is the time to finish.

Note: a laparoscopy may generate several scars, so go back and check them during later sessions until you no longer receive any response from them and they feel complete.

References

Wheeler, S. (2008). On Scar Tissue. *Structural Integration*. 36:26–30.

Wheeler, S., Blessitt, K., and Ennis, R. (2015). Integrating scar tissue into the fascial web. *Journal of Bodywork and Movement Therapies*. 19(4): 669–70.

Influencing scar tissue with movement interventions

Box 9.4 Working on scars with movement
Wojciech Cackowski

Human architecture is a creation that has so many levels of complication and depths, it is still a mystery how exactly this amazing design works. The biotensegrity model of this architectural organization shows us how complicated and extraordinary the system is and how far we are from a full understanding of human biomechanics. Models we have now are still very basic versions of all the potential possibilities and relationships within the human form.

When we think about a tensegrity as a system closed and complete in itself, which is always moving as a whole and spreading forces through the compressive and tensional elements of its architecture, we see how every movement will involve all elements of this structure, and that all of them not only need to move but to change position in relation to each other. There is also universal internal movement when we move our body. Structures, we know from the anatomy books, change their shape and position in relation to each other, thus allowing our tensegrity system to adapt to change in relation to gravity and internal/external forces. When we move, everything moves: muscles, tendons, nerves and vessels glide within their fascial sheets; muscle bellies change their shape, apparently getting thinner in elongation and bulging in contraction; organs move over each other and bones change their spatial organization, thus pulling on everything that is connected to them. The denser elements of fascial organization move in relation to other dense structures within their looser fascial

continued

organization, and the microvacuolar extracellular matrix allows for changes in the shape of all these structures.

When we have scar tissue that we would like to beneficially influence through movement, we need to ask how we can bring back the freedom of intrinsic movement needed for us to move our bones and soft tissues. Movement intervention, from a mechanical perspective and correctly used, can influence the organization of scar tissue and the inevitable restriction of our movement in a way that will restore natural soft tissue mobility to that area. We can create these restorative forces when we challenge a scarred area with a little local compression or tension that nevertheless allows it to stay within its comfort zone. This would be a starting position.

When the scar tissue becomes a little challenged by tension or compression, we can then start to mobilize this area via more distal movements. During such movements, the scarred area gets a little more or a little less challenged according to the directional forces, but the mobilization also creates different depths and directions of pull, around or towards the scarred area. This kind of approach to movement intervention has been developed specifically for rebalancing those regions of the body affected by fascial restrictions, one cause of which may be scars and adhesions.

Guidelines for working on scars with movement
These moves should only be practised once a scar is well-healed, and should not be painful. Work slowly with awareness and focus on how your body is reacting; the movements should feel good. The body should feel more free and fluid afterwards, not sore or tired. When done with care, all these movements are safe.

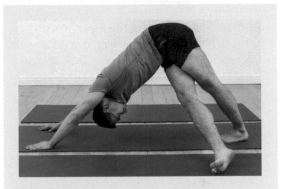

Figure 9.5
Downward facing dog.

In Figure 9.5, observe how by using downward facing dog and adopting different strategies of movement then from this starting point one can move in a compression strategy for abdominal scarring. Bend the knees, bringing them up towards the abdomen and chest opposite the shoulders. Twist the pelvis in relation to the shoulders. Bend the elbows and bring the chest towards the legs. By folding lumbar spine into flexion with a posterior tilt of the pelvis, you can create folding and separation through compression in the abdominal area that will promote separation of the adhered layers in the abdominal area.

Figure 9.6 demonstrates a variation on downward facing dog by taking one leg away, thus creating greater shearing forces along the abdominal layers.

In Figure 9.7 you can see a change in strategy, which pulls tissues from above the pelvis towards the lower extremities. Fixing the upper body on the floor and creating a pull on the tissues from below by leg movement creates a downward pull on tissues, and through

continued

different movements of the leg will create several different vectors pulling in a downward direction, helping to mobilize tissues downwards towards a scar in the abdominal area.

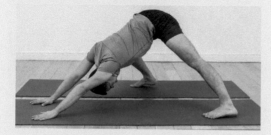

Figure 9.6
A variation on downward facing dog.

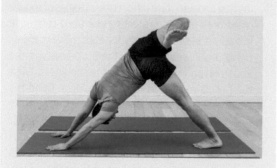

Figure 9.7
Pulling tissues from above the pelvis towards the lower extremities.

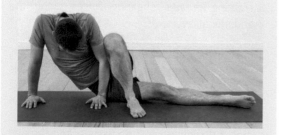

Figure 9.8

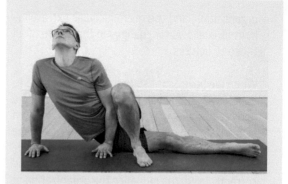

Figure 9.9

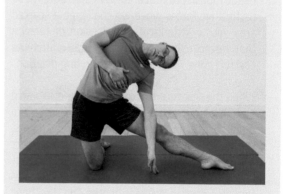

Figure 9.10

Figures 9.8-9.10 demonstrate other strategies for creating different tensional relationships between deeper and more superficial layers around the abdominal area. When the surface is tensioned on one side, the other side is relaxed and pulled into a more local tensional relationship by spinal movements of extension and flexion, which creates a different pull on the surface compared with the deeper pull exerted by the other side.

Assessing and treating your client   *Chapter* 10

Jan Trewartha

Introduction

This chapter could feasibly be titled "Assessing and treating a scar", but by now it should be clear that a scar is so much more than the visible mark left by surgery or an accident. As we have seen, even the tiniest, least visible scar can have global effects and, when assessing a client, we need to look at them "in the macro and the micro" to ensure that we understand, as much as is possible, the three-dimensional ramifications. This involves looking at:

- The scar itself, its history, how it was created and how it has healed.

- Adhesions from the scar – where they link to and what effect they might be having.

- The full body; posture, gait, and compensation patterns.

- Anomalies, for example, in proprioception and the neurovascular system.

- How the scar affects the client emotionally.

We have seen how damage in one part of the body can have local and distal effects on function and mobility, but how does this inform how we, as therapists, work? We start to comprehend that if scar tissue has certain consequences, then changing that tissue must have pro rata results. Crumple a tea-towel in one corner and the folds will radiate out to the edges; let go and the material can be shaken back into its normal shape. We stop seeing the body as a series of parts; traditional anatomy textbooks isolate structures and organs, but this is not representative of our living bodies in which everything is connected to everything else and it is impossible to operate on, injure or heal any part of the body without body-wide effects. This concept of "body-wide" must then be translated from the traditional linear view into the multidimensional if we are to truly grasp the potential ramifications of any injury or scarring. And then of what local tissue healing might, considering the multiple determining factors, in its turn achieve globally.

Listen to the client

How is your client affected by their scar(s)? We have already looked at the emotions generated around scars (Chapter 8), so we know it is important to allow someone to talk about how they feel (if they wish to). We must be aware that emotions and memories may surface and should be listened to with respect. As therapists, part of our work is to "hold the space", a term used for providing a safe and nurturing environment for our clients. Being with them quietly, letting them know we can stop working if they wish, and having paper tissues at hand should they be needed: this is all part of our job and should be carried out with as little interjection as possible to avoid interrupting the process they are going through.

Elicit the history of the scar

- Operation or injury?

- Reason/cause?

- Type and approach?

- Elective or emergency surgery? (Level of shock experienced.)

- Infected or inflamed at the time? (Tracking adhesions may be present.)

- Drain/cannula/scope sites? (Tracking adhesions may be present.)

- Tenderness or pain?

- Repaired under emergency conditions? (This may affect the quality of the suturing.)

- Scar well-healed?

For a hip/knee replacement or similar, for how long had the client been waiting for surgery? This will affect the level of physical compensation that is evident. This should then be addressed, ideally in parallel with the scar treatment, using fascia release therapies to free the myofascial holding patterns.

Visual and manual assessment of the scar

Please note that assessments should be performed with your client in minimal clothing, e.g., underwear, in order to provide a clear picture of the body.

An experienced therapist will often be able to tell where the restriction is in their client's body as they walk into the room. It can take years of practice to reach that point. Body reading is a very useful skill and below follow some guidelines of what to look for in any client, with particular reference to a client with a scar.

The most obvious imbalances can stem from the abdomen and pelvis; deep, internal adhesions may cause abdominal or pelvic rotation, and this is usually evident if you draw an imaginary gravity line from nose to navel, down to the to symphysis pubis to between their feet (ask the client to march on the spot for a few steps to ensure the feet are in their natural position first). Deviation from that line may be an indicator of internal torsion, although there are other possible causes such as restrictions in the lumbar area or in the psoas. You will have access to the client's full medical history to help you with your assessment. Whatever the different possible contributing factors, scarring may be one of them.

Two examples of internal torsion

In Figure 10.1, note that the client leans slightly to her left, and yet the tissues are pulling to the right between the navel and the appendectomy scar, demonstrating internal distortion. It is interesting to see that in the "after" photo (Figure 10.1B), the situation has already started to change after only one hour of work. The improved tautness of the upper abdomen is clear, and linearity has returned to what was previously a distorted cholecystectomy scar. The navel is more open, the client is standing straighter, the tissue pull is hugely reduced, and in general the skin texture looks to have improved.

Figures 10.2 A and B show a less dramatic situation featuring a history of appendectomy

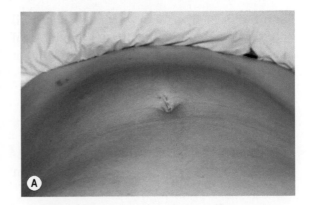

Figure 10.2A
Abdomen congested and pulling to the client's right.

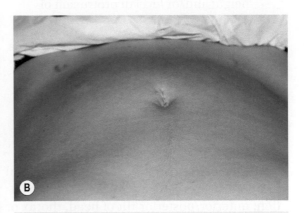

Figure 10.2B
Two hours later, following work by supervised students, the abdomen is more defined and central. "Before the treatment, I had a constant pulling sensation from my appendix scar and below my belly button. I no longer have that pulling sensation and my belly button has opened up to the size it was before the laparoscopies. Things feel much freer and more comfortable now."

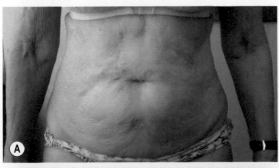

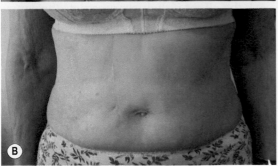

Figure 10.1
(A) Before and (B) after one hour of treatment on the cholecystectomy scar (vertical linear) and appendectomy scar.

and multiple laparoscopy scars: a slight pull of the navel to the right with poor abdominal definition, and post-treatment improvement are demonstrated.

Standing assessment

Look for signs of internal torsion and of imbalance. These may include differences when comparing:

- left and right sternocleidomastoid tension
- shoulder height
- height and/or level of protrusion of scapulae
- "fat creases" of lower thoracic/waist area
- hip height
- level of hands against legs and angle of rotation.

You should also look out for: medial/lateral rotation of legs and feet; pronation/supination; anterior/posterior tilt of head, thorax or pelvis; head angled to one side; and scoliosis, kyphosis or lordosis.

Make comprehensive notes – it helps to sketch your findings onto A4 paper with a body outline showing front, back and side views to give you a visual sense of what is happening for your client. Mark the scar(s) on the outline. Use curving arrows to demonstrate lines of internal torsion. Feel for areas of tension and congestion and mark them down as well: what feels normal and what feels wrong? Feedback from your client will assist you.

Walking assessment

Your client walks away then back to you slowly. At the point of turning around, the client should stop for a second to rebalance before walking back to you: this makes for a clearer analysis. You are looking for the following: leaning to one side; limping; limited foot flexion; foot drag, lateral/medial rotation of feet; leading with one leg; walking sideways (crab-like); prominent or varicose veins in the legs; popliteal congestion; uneven arm swing; an inability to walk in a straight line (proprioceptive disruption). Also ask the client if they have any areas of their body that feel numb or hypersensitive.

Range of movement

Ask the client if their scar restricts their movement and, if so, to demonstrate how. You can video or photograph the issue, but remember that there is room for variation in a clinic situation and a client's feedback after receiving scar therapy is more convincing proof of the efficacy of treatment, unless (for example) you can obtain a video-recording of their gait before and after, demonstrating an obvious improvement.

Comparing left with right and palpating with your hands once your client is on the therapy couch helps to confirm what you think are seeing (Figure 10.3).

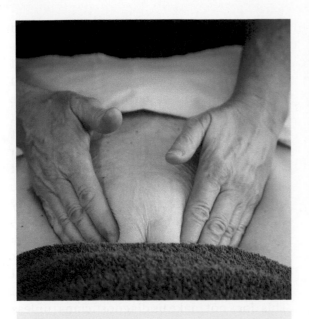

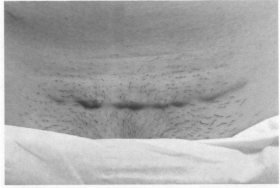

Figure 10.4
An example of a hypertrophic scar.

Figure 10.3
When comparing left and right anywhere on the body, keep your hands evenly positioned at the same angle to ensure accurate comparison.

Photo credit: Adam Trewartha

Hypertrophic scar

Collagen production has not ceased when it should, but the raised, often reddened and thickened scar is confined to the original scar boundary (Figure 10.4).

Keloid scar

"An abnormal scar that forms at the site of an injury or an incision and spreads beyond the borders of the original lesion...[A] swirling mass of collagen fibers and fibroblasts... Common features include thickened, raised, itchy clusters of scar tissue...and are often red or darker in color than surrounding skin. Keloids occur when the body continues to produce the tough, fibrous collagen after a wound has healed" (Keeney Smith and Ryan 2016). Keloids tend to be sensitive and can be extremely disfiguring. They are more common in people with higher levels

Scar typing

Every scar is unique. Literature on the grading of scars is available, but that is not the focus of this book. However, it is important to know whether a scar is keloid or hypertrophic because no abrasive technique should ever be used on these raised scars as they will often redden and become tender. Work around such scars, not on them. This also applies to grafts and burns while in a fragile state, until some resilience has developed.

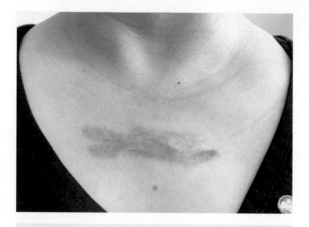

Figure 10.5
This scar started as half the size of a pea as a result of a chickenpox rash, but painful cortisone injections led to it spreading. The client would cover the scar, but the irritation and sensitivity were severe. She says: "After the treatment I cried my eyes out. I felt emotionally released. I felt that my left-sided neck and shoulder tension that I've always put down as tension from working, released. I felt lighter, happier and pain-free. Since then, I've hardly touched my scar. I look at it and I am not embarrassed by it anymore. I now see it as part of me and the most important thing for me is that I don't disassociate myself from it anymore. I have not covered it or hidden it since." (Also see Chapter 8).

of pigmentation in their skin (of Asian, Afro-Caribbean and Hispanic origin) and appear primarily on earlobes, upper chest, arms/shoulders, head and neck, but can appear anywhere (Figure 10.5).

Palpation
The art of palpation

Palpation is a skill that is acquired not just from going on a course, but from years of practice. Learning how the body should feel can also be helped by attending dissection courses; this helps us envisage what is under our hands and to understand full body relationships, particularly when the course is biotensegrity-informed. Knowing the feel of the body is vital for a therapist, but those with less experience will benefit from simply comparing left with right throughout (Figure 10.3), and this provides good, basic information. Being aware of how a body should feel – its tensions, textures, temperature, density, responsiveness and tissue mobility – we automatically start to pick up what feels wrong, even with no medical background or years of practice behind us. This does not make us diagnosticians (unless we have the appropriate training), but it will develop our sensory feedback to a higher level. It also makes it easier to tell, when we are working, whether the tissue is responding or not. Lewit and Olsanka (2004) noted that a great advantage of manual techniques is that the hand is an instrument that senses, establishing such a feedback relationship.

Palpating the scar and surrounding area

Gently palpate the area with both hands, searching for hot or cold, for hardened, over-soft or non-resilient tissue (with lack of bounce), and tissue pull. Drop deeper into the surrounding tissues, keeping your elbows bent to ensure that you are not pushing – that is a very different action – feeling for areas of tenderness, numbness, congestion/density and hardness; follow to see if they link into proximal organs, bones or joints.

In Chapter 3 we saw how deep fascial layers may not be fully sutured in an emergency situation. Place your fingers along the scar and allow them to drop into any tissue "gap". Unless tissue has been removed, for example, as in excision of a tumor or lipoma, the apparently missing tissue can often be gently encouraged through the Scraping technique (see Chapter 9, pp. 122–123) to "go home" before the surgically induced layers are then integrated with the Matching Layers technique to create a more resilient tissue (see Chapter 9, p. 123); the client often feels more connected, particularly in the case of cesarean (C-section) repairs (see Chapter 11, pp. 145–147, for a C-section case study).

Check the tissue tension, noting that the skin will not stretch as far as normal when a scar is adhered to underlying structures (Figure 10.6).

Check what proximal structures a restriction may be affecting (Figure 10.7).

Next, feel for irregularities along the length of the scar and around it, indicating sites of congestion or adhesion (Figure 10.8).

Spend time assessing the scar and the effect it appears to be having proximally and distally. In laparoscopic surgery, the damage may be obvious some distance from the wound sites, where the surgical procedure itself took place, and where the surgeon has "scoped" during the operation.

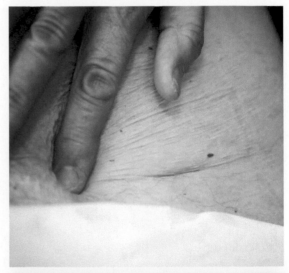

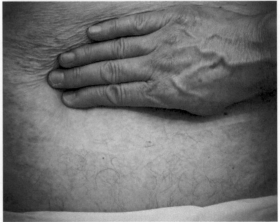

Figure 10.6
Checking the tissue tension around the scar.

Photo credit: Adam Trewartha

As you drop deeper into the tissues around the scar, palpating and assessing, feel for congestion which may be due to adhesions, always remaining alert to other possible

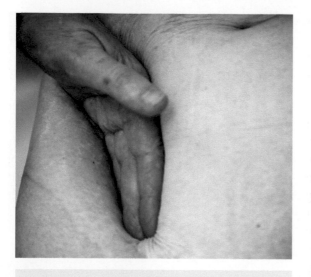

Figure 10.7
Checking to see whether the right iliac crest and anterior superior iliac spine (ASIS) are restricted by adhesions from a C-section scar. Be aware that other causative factors may be associated with such limitations, not just adhesions.

Photo credit: Adam Trewartha

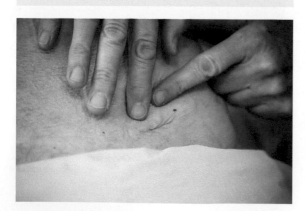

Figure 10.8
Assessing the scar and its surrounding area.

Photo credit: Adam Trewartha

causes: Lewit and Olsanka (2004) pointed out that when working with scars by manually engaging with the "barrier" created by internal adhesions: "just as with other soft tissue… we obtain release after a short latency, almost without increasing pressure." If we do not and "the resistance does not change" then a pathology may be present (Figure 10.9). This highlights the absolute necessity of engaging with and following the tissues, and not imposing our demands upon them.

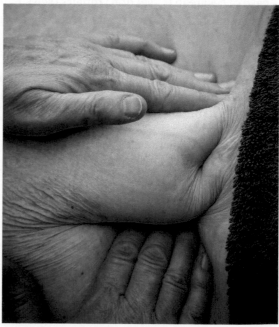

Figure 10.9
Manually engaging with a barrier discovered on palpation. This is gentle, and therefore comfortable for the client; if this is due to adhesions, release after a short latency would be expected.

Photo credit: Adam Trewartha

Fourie and Sharkey (2018) point out that different nationalities, weather, nutrition, collagen patterns and mindsets can affect the body and how the fascia feels on palpation. Again, comparing left and right correctly (Figure 10.3) will, regardless of these factors, allow the therapist to effectively assess that particular client and their scar.

In all scars, look closely at the polyhedral pattern of the skin: it may be distorted or flattened. Hair growth may be affected around the scar. The skin may also be shiny rather than matte.

Finally, ask the client to feel the scar before you start work – in many cases they will not have touched it for years (if ever). I always feel reasonably confident that the scar will feel different after about 10 minutes of ScarWork[1]. I ask the client to feel the scar again when it starts to change and several times throughout the treatment so that they can feel part of the process, engaging with the scar. This also helps their emotional reintegration with that part of their body.

Developing your sensitivity and awareness

Some people have an innate sensitivity, and some need practice to develop it. There

follows a simple exercise to help you develop your awareness when working with bodies in general, as well as with scars. Restrictions are not only due to scarring and adhesions, after all. Muscular contractions, pathologies and emotional tension: these are just some of the possible reasons why the therapist might feel a dragging, a tension, a tissue densification. In this case, the restriction created by the index finger of one person represents the scar, and the therapist senses where that scar is using both hands but keeping their eyes closed. To make it

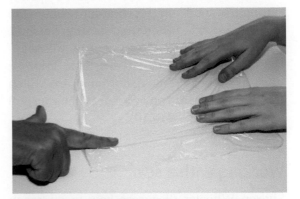

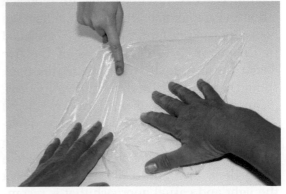

Figure 10.10

Identifying the vectors of pull from the point of restriction.

---

1 Where the term "ScarWork" is used, this refers to Sharon Wheeler's ScarWork. The term "scar therapy", where used, refers generally to any modality addressing scar tissue.

more challenging, place a coin, or even a hair, under the cling-film (plastic wrap) and try to locate it. You can add more sheets of cling-film to create density or depth.[2]

Use sheets of ready-perforated, plastic cling-film. Two people are needed for this exercise. Person 1, who is sensing, places their hands lightly on the bottom of the cling-film and shuts their eyes. Person 2 puts one finger somewhere else on the cling-film and leaves it there. Person 1 now has to sense, by gently testing the "pull" on the cling-film, where the holding finger is. When they are sure, Person 1 tries to touch the holding fingertip, still keeping their eyes closed. The test is to improve one's awareness of the distortion point, which then translates into an awareness of tissue pull in the body (Figure 10.10).

Working with a scar

Sharon Wheeler discusses how to approach a scar in Chapter 9. It is important to note the contraindications for ScarWork, also provided in Chapter 9. The descriptions of the five ScarWork techniques we offer in this book should be used with the accompanying videos. (Scan the QR code on page 121 to access them.) These will help you make at least some difference to many of the scars you encounter. Please read the contraindications carefully before using these techniques. Their names reflect the light and casual approach that is recommended to get the best results from ScarWork.

Personally, I work on the scars before giving any other treatment. It seems common sense that this helps to de-tension the system, which then facilitates more effective restoration of normal balance in the body.

Crossed scars

A scar generally heals less effectively when it is part of two scars crossing or a T-junction. Where two or more scars cross or meet in a T, the skin has been cut in two directions; at the point where the scars meet it is more difficult to align the fibers. Hence, the crossing tends to be an area that, although helped by scar therapy, often does not always resolve as well as the other scars (Figure 10.11).

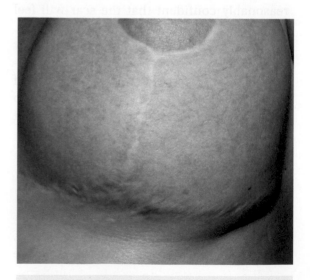

Figure 10.11
Breast augmentation scar.

---

2   This exercise is reproduced by kind permission of Fourie, W., and Sharkey, J. (2018).

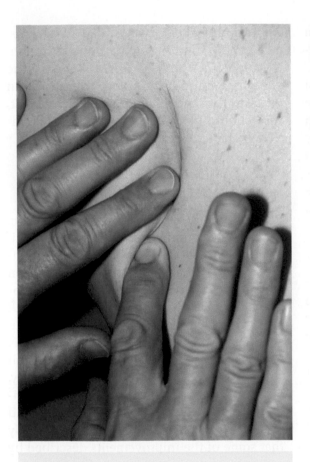

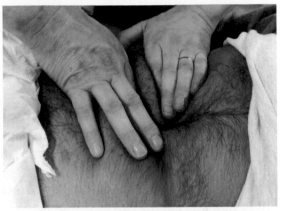

Figure 10.13
Following the tissue working on abdominal adhesions. Never force or push but trust the body. This work looks strong, but it is not: it is simply tissue-led and very comfortable for the client.

Figure 10.12
When working with a scar, allow the tissue to lead you.

Follow the tissue!

Like a woman learning to follow her dance partner, a therapist has to learn to follow the tissue. Imposing our own demands because we think tissue should go in a certain direction is not useful. "Tissue goes home" is the mantra, and any attempts to override this natural tendency can limit the healing potential – or even create further damage. If you are unable to feel where the tissue wants to go, use the exercise provided earlier in this chapter to develop your sensitivity, and then practice it with friends. Consistent feedback from your client to ensure that there is no pain or discomfort will indicate that you are working within the safety guidelines. When the tissue is transforming in this way, it should feel right and good to both the client and the therapist. Thus, you will know you are working with the body and not against it. If the client does not feel comfortable then stop what you are doing, change your approach and, primarily, use an even lighter touch (Figures 10.12 and 10.13).

The importance of integration
(see also Appendices I and II)

The concept of this book is to demonstrate our innate connectivity and flow, that is, the body working as one integrated system, and the tissue continuity enabling adaptation and optimized function. Scars and adhesions disrupt that continuity, and adhesions connect structures which should not be connected. When scar therapies reduce these artificial connections, the body can still demonstrate long-held compensatory myofascial patterning. Fascia-based therapies facilitate this freeing of restriction and restoration of connectivity. As the planes of tissue that were stuck together become unstuck, fluid flow and gliding can be restored.

Not only does reintegration need to occur at the physical level, but it also needs to take place on an emotional level. A scar that disfigures, disables or hurts can make us feel negative towards it (see Chapter 8). We can become disengaged from a part of our body if it is no longer attractive or functional. "This leg is holding me back!" "If only I could move this arm – it's useless!" Whole-body integration will help to restore physical sensation and mentally enable a client to reconnect with the scar site. I find that clients often say "I feel like me again" after ScarWork, and integration complements the treatment by helping to restore a sense of whole-body connection. "Gentle touch may impact the mechanotransduction pathways to release the tension associated with scar retraction and induce apoptosis of myofibroblasts, leading to softening and integration of the scarring within the body in both the physiological and psychological sense" (Box 8.1, Chapter 8, pp. 108–109). Therefore, after giving any kind of scar therapy, allow time to work with the whole body.

Appendices I and II at the end of this chapter give simple ways of facilitating integration. If you are not trained in fascial work and the client is seen to have severe compensation patterns that continue after your treatment, they should be referred to a suitably qualified practitioner.

Recording the results

Photograph the scar and the surrounding area, and also video any anomalies in gait or range of movement before and after treatment. Some of my best results have been experienced by clients who I forgot to photograph, or where I thought it was just a small scar which would therefore not show up significantly in a photograph. For example, on a course, students took the photograph shown in Figure 10.14; it is not good quality, but even in actuality the scar was scarcely visible. Had we included the lower face, neck and shoulders, anterior and posterior, it is likely that some of the improvements described by

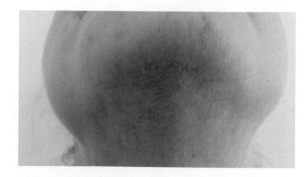

Figure 10.14
A near-invisible scar under the chin.

the client would have been obvious in the before-and-after treatment comparison.

Pre-treatment, this scar had been considered by the client to be non-problematic. Here is her feedback:

"History of scar: injury occurred during a swimming lesson over 40 years ago, landing chin and head on the edge of a swimming pool. Wound was left open for approximately four hours with lower jaw exposed before being stitched together with 10 stitches.

During: I felt sensations of emotional release when work was done in the middle section of the scar. Feelings of short "zaps" throughout the treatment. Lower lip released, although there were no visible signs of restriction on the lip, the release felt like the lip smiling widely.

After: freer movement of the area below the lower lip, less "attached". Neck rotation much easier with less crunching. Scar feels smoother and wire-like line almost negligible. Distance between neck and shoulders feels extended and relaxed."

Feedback from the client, not only immediately after the treatment but a few weeks later, will validate what you believe you have accomplished. During the subsequent two to three weeks, certainly after ScarWork and probably after other light touch scar therapies, the body appears to carry on changing, as though the work has triggered a healing process that is automatically continued. There may be visual and internal changes that were not apparent after the session. Therefore, leave three weeks between treatment sessions for this very reason.

Ease of reference for the therapist

We are all used to comprehensively recording a client's medical history. When working on scars, it is helpful also to have a visual reference, especially with multiple scarring. If, as recommended earlier, you use a body outline to record your assessment, this allows you to mark the positions of scars and make notes regarding their origin and effect. (Most scars are worked on several times, unless they are small and responsive, when one treatment may be enough). The date each scar was treated should also be marked for ease of reference, and adding a tick indicates that the work on a scar is now complete. Arrows can be used to indicate torsion patterns and tissue pull (remember that the latter may not only be scar-related, but could also be linked with other historical injuries or with behavioral patterns).

Client reaction

It is possible a client might feel mistrustful of the light touch approach, especially if they believe that scars need to be "broken down" by a strong hand. Understanding the power of light touch (see Chapter 5) will enable you to be confident in your approach and to help ease the client's fears. Rule number 1 is not to go heavier to gain more effect; if you do not appear to be changing the tissue then go lighter and lighter. This may be counterintuitive, and the client may not understand this initially, but scars respond best to a light, casual and relaxed touch; once you have tried this and felt the tissue transform under your fingers, you will see the body differently, and consequently your client will learn to trust this approach.

Appendix I: Integration

Integration is performed by therapists to settle, connect and ground a client, and also to minimize any possible discomfort after treatment.

As we have seen, when addressing scars we are working not only locally but also body-wide. The adhesions beneath the surface may well be affecting the myofascia globally, and thus it is important after treatment to enable the body to process the interventions as much as possible. This limits the discomfort that may otherwise be felt by the client and assists them in letting go, both physically and emotionally.

N.B. Do not underestimate the amount of time it takes to fully integrate the body after scar therapy has been given. Allow at least 20 minutes. This book has demonstrated the potential ramifications and effects of scars; integration allows for vital structural re-balancing after the treatment. If the client has severe postural/compensation issues due to scarring and/or other causes, then further fascial work is probably indicated. If you are untrained, then you must refer the client to an appropriate therapist.

You may be used to working with integration but, if not, you could adopt the following procedure. Use a relaxed, very light touch. Put one hand very lightly over the area worked upon and the other farther away; for example, across the pelvis after working on a C-section scar, then down the legs to reconnect, as women often feel "cut in two" after a C-section (Figure 10.15). Ensure balance is maintained by working on both sides of the body. One technique puts one hand underneath the client and the other hand on top, sandwiching the area, and ensuring that you can sense a continuity between your hands.

Be comfortable as you stand/sit there, breathing calmly, with your focus on reconnecting the different areas of the body as you work with them. That is all you need to do. For example, if someone has had a particularly unpleasant leg injury then their natural response may be anger, as well as dislike of the scars and of the leg itself. Acceptance of the scar by the client will happen naturally when the scars become less ugly, but you can help that process by using this technique. If the approach is somewhat alien to you then it may be tempting to dismiss it completely, but do try it with an open mind and ask for client feedback to validate what you might feel while working: the client may be able to feel more than you can and this will help you develop your own awareness and confidence.

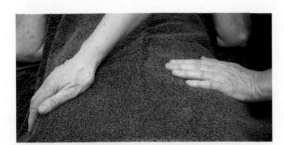

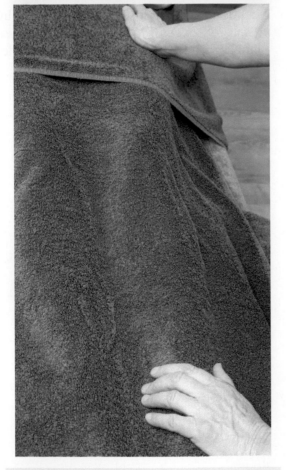

Appendix II: Occipito-sacral balancing

This is a cranio-sacral technique. It aims to restore/maintain normal connectivity within the spine.

With the client prone, supine (if light-weight) or lying on their side, place one hand gently on the occiput and one on the sacrum (Figure 10.16).

Rest lightly and have the intention of restoring flow. You may, after a few moments, feel as though one hand is being "filled", almost as if something is expanding beneath it. Then the flow will move up/down the spine and the other hand will feel filled. Or you may feel a pulse at each end. The flow will be at 6-12 cycles per minute.

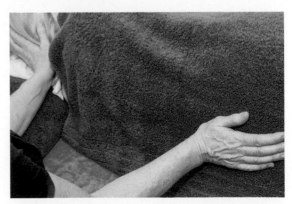

Figure 10.15
Integration after C-section treatment; the lighter your hands, the better the results.

Photo credit: Adam Trewartha

Figure 10.16
Occipito-sacral balancing; use the lightest of touches, not putting pressure on the body.

Photo credit: Adam Trewartha

Even if you do not feel the flow beneath your hands, if you hold the occipito-sacral position for about five minutes then the body will use the touch to its benefit. For more details on cranio-sacral methods, see Parsons and Marcer (2006).

References

Fourie, W., and Sharkey, J. (2018). S.C.A.R Therapy Workshop. Edinburgh Training & Conference Venue, Edinburgh, UK, 25–26 June 2018.

Keeney Smith, N., and Ryan, C. (2016). *Traumatic Scar Tissue Management*, page 87. Edinburgh, UK: Handspring Publishing.

Lewit, K., and Olsanka, S. (2004). Clinical importance of active scars: abnormal scars as a cause of myofascial pain. *Journal of Manipulative and Physiological Therapeutics.* 27:399–402.

Parsons, J., and Marcer, N. (2006). Osteopathy: *models for diagnosis, treatment and practice.* Edinburgh, UK: Churchill Livingston, Elsevier.

Case studies

Jan Trewartha

Chapter 11

Introduction

In this chapter we will look at three documented case studies of varying levels of complexity. The first one demonstrates results achieved through using just two of the techniques we offer you in the videos linked to this book (scan the QR code on page 121 to access the videos); a gentle, light treatment combined with integration provided a quick and a rewarding result. The second and third studies are more complex.

It is easy to feel pressured to produce results when a client walks in, in a traumatized state, as illustrated in the third case study. ScarWork is most effective when given with a gentle, relaxed and casual touch, almost with an attitude of "I wonder what will happen?" The easy, descriptive names of the techniques deliberately reflect this approach. During the third case study, there was a lot of laughter: there was no other way as Bella was in such dire straits. With the humor, the care and the joy of being touched gently, her body responded slowly but surely. Such an approach, combined with empathy, is one that generally works well for therapists, rather than being determined to get someone better against all odds; we are, in the end, not there to fix people but to be catalysts, assisting them as they return themselves to health.

Case study 1: Treatment of scar following excision of malignant melanoma

A 48-year-old woman presented with emotional issues and recent difficulties in concentrating on her work as an accountant (which she had previously enjoyed), following the death of her husband the previous year.

> **Box 11.1** Medical history and general health
>
> - 7 years earlier: excision of mole on the right side of her throat.
> - 6 years earlier: lymph node biopsy (same region).
> - 5 years earlier: excision of malignant melanoma and stage 3 lymph gland carcinoma (same region). Road traffic accident with probable neck whiplash.
> - 5 months earlier: started Emotional Freedom Therapy (EFT) to resolve the deep grief that remained after her bereavement but was unsure of how much benefit had been received.

The client reported that she felt good (apart from underlying grief) with 10/10 energy level. She undertook regular sporting activity. Her diet consisted of freshly cooked food

143

and had a high fruit and vegetable content; she consumed no alcohol, and her coffee and tea intake was low; she drank less than one liter of water daily. She had experienced three pregnancies with two live births (one with ventouse suction).

Treatment

After examination, it was considered likely that adhesions had developed between the original scar and the sternocleidomastoid muscle, and that there was also possible involvement with the jugular vein, hyoid bone and various fascial tissues.

This client had a 1.5 hour session of Scar-Work, in which the ScarWork techniques Feather Light Sweeping (FLS) and Down the Rabbit Hole (DTRH) were used (Figure 11.1). Because she felt distraught with grief, a lot of treatment time was spent on integration and relaxation to help her on an emotional as well as a physical level.

During the DTRH part of the treatment, she could feel a tracking sensation underneath the scar, and continued to feel a sense of movement in this region for the next few weeks "as though it was readjusting itself".

After treatment, the client experienced an excruciating headache "like the worst migraine ever", one she felt was similar to that which had occurred after the

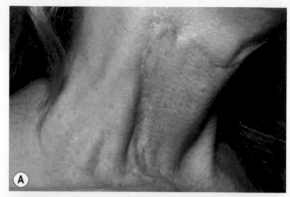
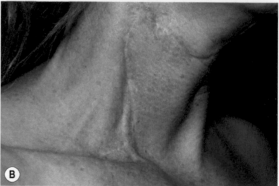

Figure 11.1

(A) The post-operative throat scar that followed the excision of a malignant melanoma and stage 3 lymph gland carcinoma; (B) the same scar after 1.5 hours of treatment showing a change in surface contours.

surgery. Although she occasionally experienced migraines, she reported that this one was much more severe than usual; it was eventually relieved by analgesia.

During a follow-up discussion, the client stated that the treatment had: "done far more than any 1.5 hour treatment should". And not only physically, but also emotionally.

"After the surgery I was much less of a talker, something I have been doing incessantly all my life, and in fact rather than speaking out, I had let resentments in my marriage build up over time with no outlet. In the first few weeks after the treatment, however, I noticed that I miraculously found words to express my feelings." (See also Chapter 8).

Case study 2: Treatment of cesarean scar

A 40-year-old woman presented with low thoracic back pain and incontinence issues. Two cesarean births had left a scar with a ridge above it, and aching, numbness and a feeling of hardness in this region (Figure 11.2).

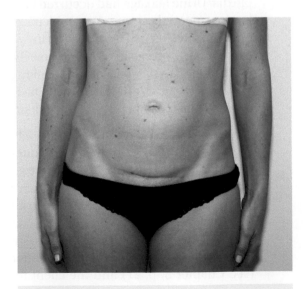

Figure 11.2
Before treatment, the client demonstrated a marked torso tilt to the left.

Box 11.2 Medical history and general health

- Other scars: episiotomy and epidural from first birth.
- Excision of moles on face, chest and abdomen.
- Extreme urinary urgency, especially when jogging. If rectum is full then the urgency is almost uncontrollable. When she urinates, there is incomplete emptying of the bladder.
- Experiences occasional mild stress incontinence. Anxiety when she feels the need to open her bowels as does not feel confident of full bowel control.
- Lower thoracic back pain from "two to three years" prior to consultation.
- Feeling of "lump in throat" since second birth 4.5 years earlier, when a strong feeling of pulsing in the solar plexus, which seemed connected with the throat, started.
- Eight pregnancies with three live births (two terminations and three miscarriages). First birth vaginal and traumatic, with epidural and episiotomy followed by sessions of specialist physiotherapy and pelvic floor exercises. Sexual intercourse was not possible for one year after the birth. Planned C-sections for her other two births.
- 80% conductive hearing loss developed after the pregnancies – artificial replacement of stapes bone in ear.
- No other relevant history. The client walks and jogs regularly, generally eats healthily but can lapse into bad habits; she drinks adequate fluids and has a high energy level.

Chapter 11

Examination

The C-scar felt ridged along its edges. Tension from the scar fed into the right hip, and the client remembered that she always carried her babies on that hip (see Chapter 3, pp. 24–25 on postural adaptation). Palpation revealed discomfort in the upper central abdomen and around the C-scar.

Treatment

Three 1.5-hour treatments were given over two- to three-week intervals. Integration work was given after each session.

1. FLS[1] was employed for 30 minutes until general softening of the C-scar and abdomen was achieved. The client reported "something releasing" in her lumbar back and also feeling more relaxed. DTRH[2] was applied to the mole excision scars.

2. After the first treatment, the usual low thoracic pain was followed by additional aching in the left groin and buttock, which continued for five days. (Advice is always given to avoid heavy strain on the body for at least three days post-treatment as the internal shifts are usually ongoing, but the client had been carrying more than normal during preparations for Christmas.) Upon arrival at the clinic, there was aching in both groins and a sensation of "pins and needles" in the solar plexus region. On palpation, the C-scar felt softer with ridging unchanged, but not causing any localized discomfort. There had been no incidents of urinary urgency, although the client had not been jogging.

   Treatment: FLS[1] and Matching Layers[3] techniques, were applied to the C-scar. Once again, the client felt the lumbar area softening, and a relaxing sensation in the solar plexus.

3. The client reported improvement in back pain but some mild aching in the left hip and gluteal regions. She was still experiencing a tingling sensation in the solar plexus. Urine leakage had occurred once but in general there were no problems. That morning, she had succeeded in controlling the need to open her bowels without anxiety. There was no urgency to pass urine despite a full bowel. A fast power walk had not created an incident.

   Treatment: FLS to the C-scar. The *mons pubis* had slumped, as often happens, possibly due to the retraction pattern created during surgery. This tissue was repositioned during the session using a technique not covered in this book; an example of tissue "going home" given the right facilitation (see Chapter 3, p. 21) and the client felt

---

1 FLS, Feather Light Sweeping ScarWork technique.

2 DTRH, Down the Rabbit Hole ScarWork technique.

3 Matching Layers ScarWork technique.

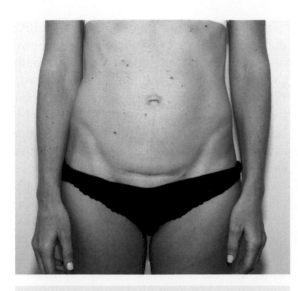

Figure 11.3
After three treatments, the client's low thoracic discomfort was still present but had lessened, and her posture had improved. Relief of incontinence had taken place. More ScarWork was still needed, while fascial work would be beneficial to correct the postural imbalance.

happy at more normal contours being re-established. Direct fascial release work helped free superficial fascial restrictions in the suprapubic, sub-clavicular regions and over the sternum. The client returned for a final photograph (Figure 11.3) two weeks after the final treatment. The scar was softer and no longer ridged. Low thoracic pain continued but had lessened. Bowel and bladder control were both hugely improved. On that particular morning, she had jogged for 35 minutes with no feeling of bladder weakness.

Summary

The C-scars and consequent adhesions could be reasonably assumed to have been affecting bowel and bladder function; treatment appeared to have improved bladder control and, to a certain extent, bowel control. As can be seen from Figure 11.3, more ScarWork could be useful and, ideally, some fascia-focused therapy to further improve structural balance.

Client feedback

Two months after her last treatment session, the client confirmed that the low thoracic pain had improved. Bladder control was also greatly improved, although she still chose to urinate more often than normal as a pre-emptive measure. Bowel control: she still experienced urgency but reported that she is "far more able and confident about controlling it than I was prior to the treatment."

She continued: "My treatment was eye-opening. I was not entirely sure what to expect when I started and after seeing a number of professionals, all offering different approaches, I was feeling pretty despondent about my various issues. This treatment for my scar was calm, gentle and, most importantly, it has been the most beneficial out of everything I have tried. It has also helped me to understand my body's working better. I'm very grateful for being lucky enough to have found this practice."

Case study 3: Infant congenital intestinal atresia

Specific medical history

When Bella was born nothing obvious was wrong, but three days later it became evident that she had ileal atresia: her bowel was not functioning and toxicity was building (no appetite, abdominal distension, no passing of feces, and evident illness). Emergency night-time admission to hospital resulted in the excision of two-thirds of the small intestine and a bowel resection, leaving a large scar in the lower left abdomen (Figure 11.4). Post-operatively there were few issues except, as she grew older, Bella complained of occasional pain after opening the bowels. She is dairy-intolerant. When Bella went through periods of growth, she also experienced bowel discomfort, which she put down to growing pains.

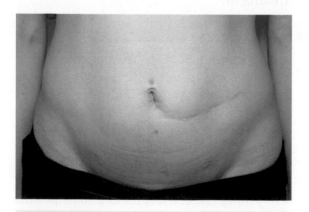

Figure 11.4
The original scar was later added to by numerous laparoscopies.

At 15 years of age, stretching up to paint a door, Bella experienced sudden, extreme bowel discomfort and was bedridden all day in pain; she was admitted to hospital for further investigation. Bowel obstruction was suspected, but five weeks of conservative management in the hospital looking at her diet and medication did not help. Next, on the basis of an MRI that showed "an incomplete, subacute, small bowel obstruction" with no identifiable cause, exploratory surgery was performed on 12 September 2010 via laparoscopy, where a subacute, incomplete obstruction was observed with multiple areas of twisting and stricture throughout the whole bowel. "Extensive but soft adhesions" were excised "to free [the] entire small bowel down to [the] ileo-cecal junction." Then 300 ml of Adept (an adhesions reduction solution for intraperitoneal administration) was given.

Discharged on 15 September, Bella was readmitted as an emergency patient on 24 September, vomiting fecal matter and experiencing severe abdominal distension. The pain was located in the right abdomen at a laparoscopy site and was worse than the pre-surgical pain. Fecal vomiting had stopped upon arrival at the hospital. A catheter was inserted due to Bella's inability to empty her bladder. She was started on intravenous morphine for pain and on anti-emetics for nausea.

On October 1, while still in hospital, Bella was prescribed an anti-spasmodic, which she still takes to the present day. Bella was put on to a low-fiber diet plan (clear liquids, moving on to low residue, then low fiber and finally a diversified [high soluble, low insoluble] fiber diet), which she still resorts to today when she develops a bowel obstruction. She stayed in hospital for another month to stabilize. In general, nowadays, Bella follows the diversified fiber diet in her daily life. If she does not, or if she becomes dehydrated, then her symptoms can return, but ever since starting ScarWork treatment the frequency of recurrence has lessened. She stayed in hospital for another month to stabilize.

2011: recurrence of the 2010 symptoms; the same surgeon diagnosed adhesions and recommended repeat surgery. November 3: laparoscopic adhesiolysis for a bowel obstruction, combined with appendectomy this time due to multiple peri-appendiceal adhesions. Again, Adept was used, one liter this time. Post-operatively, Bella developed pneumonia and sepsis; these were treated with intravenous antibiotics.

2017: Bella developed abdominal discomfort. When hungry she became instantly full after a couple of mouthfuls of food. She had diarrhea for three weeks. She continued working but was exhausted. Bella started vomiting in week 4 and was admitted to hospital with a suspected intestinal obstruction. Over four weeks her weight dropped from 62 to 55 kg. A diagnosis of severe constipation was made (with "overflow", where liquid stools leak around the blockage from higher in the bowel) along with possible partial adhesive obstruction, but no surgery was performed, and Bella was sent home. Next, she was seen by her general practitioner, as she was suffering from an inability to hold down any food or to eat any solid food without experiencing pain; at this point she was living on a clear liquid diet. She was referred for cognitive behavioral therapy in December 2017 by a pain management unit (tentatively scheduled to take place in January 2020).

2018: in January Bella was seen by a gastroenterologist consultant; her weight was now down to 51 kg. On 22 January a gastric emptying study was performed, which showed her stomach being pulled down towards the navel but functioning normally; a diagnosis of probable adhesions was made. Although Bella was referred again to the colorectal surgical team, they were reluctant to operate as this would generate more adhesions. On 6 February, a defecating proctogram showed a degree of anismus. A referral for biofeedback was made, although Bella no longer considers this to be necessary. A gastrografin enema produced inconclusive results. On 6 April, Bella started treatment with ScarWork.

Bella is a warm, happy and open-hearted woman who came for treatment at the age of 25. She had been bedridden with pain for about six months and had to be driven and helped up the stairs when she first presented at the clinic. She has a good knowledge of medical terminology due to her own history (Figure 11.5); Bella's own terms for her symptoms are listed below.

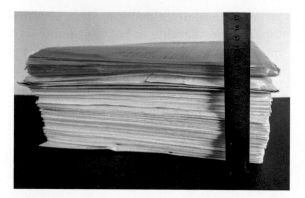

Figure 11.5
Bella's medical notes from 2010 to 2018.

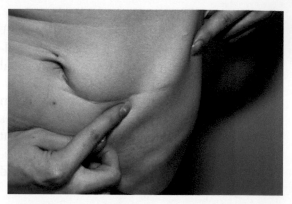

Figure 11.6
The "sausage": it changes shape and where it presents is dependent upon the location of the stool in the colon.

1. "Baby kicking": Bella feels as though she is being kicked or flicked from within. This is usually preceded by a building of pressure and discomfort and the sensation of bowel contents forcing their way through a narrowing.

2. "Vibrations": gut shakes and spasms; these can be seen externally as vibrating skin on the abdomen and to Bella feel "as though I had swallowed a mobile phone"; these vibrations were occurring every 5–15 seconds before therapy started. Upon initial consultation these were irregular with no pattern.

3. The "sausage": visible distension of lower left curve of colon when filled with stool that cannot pass. It feels as though it is stuck to and thus moves in synchronicity with the abdominal wall. It is occasionally painful but Bella continually experiences a pulling sensation. The sausage appears from above the large, left-sided surgery scar, continuing down, following the line of the colon to the pubic bone. It

changes shape and the location where it presents is dependent on where the stool is in the colon (Figure 11.6).

There was no mesh in any of the operation sites. Bella's other scars include piercings and multiple intravenous drip sites.

Box 11.3 General medical history

- 5 years old: Bella fell from her bicycle and chipped a tooth and scraped her face. No known loss of consciousness.
- 14 years old: hairline fracture, left foot.
- 14 years old: left wrist fractured in fall.
- 15 years old: all four wisdom teeth surgically removed, including a section of mandible.
- 23–24 years old: shingles.

First consultation

Bella sleeps well unless in pain, avoids all alcohol, drinks 2–3 liters of water daily and maintains a low fiber, low residue diet. She

---

Box 11.4 Medication

- Buscopan: anti-spasmodic for bowel.

- Ondansetron: anti-nausea, taken when needed.

- Mefenamic acid for menstrual pain.

- Amitriptyline: analgesia for chronic pain, previously taken daily prior to starting ScarWork treatment. Only currently taken in an emergency.

- Paracetamol and ibuprofen daily preventively for pain and inflammation.

- CBD oil multiple times daily as a fast-acting analgesic, anti-inflammatory and anti-nausea medication – "vital for managing [the] situation".

- Fresubin soya fiber easy bags. Pouches of food replacement, 500 calories each, taken orally 1–2 times daily for weight management; these help to dissolve blockages, prevent new ones, and allow the bowel to have a rest.

- Benefiber: a soluble fiber additive to food and drinks. It helps to minimize constipation, liquify stool, aid stool movement, and minimize pain and blockages.

- Multivitamins daily to counteract poor nutrient absorption.

- Probiotics after antibiotic treatment or if has a liquid stool, to restore normality.

---

reports her energy level as 0–5 out of 10 and she feels "tired, sore, worn out".

Bella's history is one of chronic pain of varying degrees throughout her life with, as documented above, three major episodes of acute and agonizing pain. She presented with abdominal distension, acute pain, swelling and hard lumps in her lower left abdomen, difficulty and pain in passing feces, foul, abnormally shaped and colored feces, and difficulty in walking. Bella experienced pain when eating solids and was on a low fiber/residue diet; between November 2017 and April 2018 she lost 19% of her body weight (62 down to 50 kg). She was unable to work or to travel independently, was in constant pain and did not know how to progress.

Ten sessions were given, three to six weeks apart. ScarWork was combined with some fascial unwinding, defined by Tozzi (2014) as: "...a dynamic functional indirect technique usually applied to the myofascial-articular complex, aimed at releasing fascial restrictions and restoration of tissue mobility and function." Integration work completed each treatment session (see Chapter 10, pp. 140–141). Abdominal torsion work was also employed for the deeper adhesions as the pain decreased over the months (Figure 11.7.); this is relatively light work which is not forceful but relies on gently following the tissue (see Chapter 10, p. 137), as does the direct fascial release technique used. At no point during any of this work should it cause pain to the client, and Bella

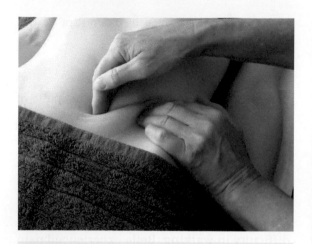

Figure 11.7
Gentle abdominal torsion work, which must be comfortable for the client, helps to clear deeper restrictions.

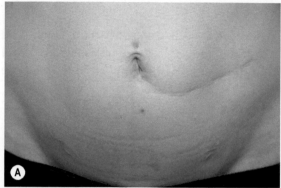

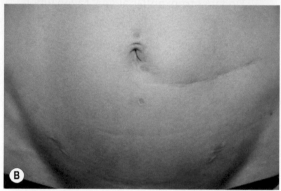

Figure 11.8
Despite only minor visible changes between the photographs taken on (A) the first and (B) last day of the case study period, the results have been profound.

was asked to report discomfort so that the pressure level could be adapted accordingly. See the treatment summary table (Table 11.1) for details of each session and outcomes. The results were primarily functional rather than aesthetic (Figure 11.8).

Summary

Bella suffered from severe adhesions from her multiple surgeries, to the point that surgeons refused further operations as more adhesions would have been created.

The course of treatment would appear to have helped to free up some of the adhesions, giving Bella back a good degree of independence, the ability to drive and to think about her future career.

Her therapy continues and she is still making good progress. At the time of writing she has moved into a flat and is independent for the first time since 2017. She has begun to drive again, can move about much more and so can see her friends. The range of food available to Bella has increased hugely; this has improved her energy levels although heavy lifting is still difficult. Her analgesia intake has been greatly reduced and a general feeling of hope for the future has been restored.

Table 11.1 Summary of Bella's treatments and results

Treatment	Treatment summary	Treatment summary report of result of treatment (obtained during follow-up session)
1	Even a light touch to Bella's abdomen was extremely uncomfortable, so Feather Light Sweeping (FLS) was employed for 30 minutes, working in from the ribs, sides and anterior iliac crests towards the center of the abdomen to calm the nerve response. Eventually, she could tolerate gentle touch to the abdomen without discomfort. Once the abdomen was calmer, the laparoscopy scars were approached using Down the Rabbit Hole technique (DTRH). DTRH is very light touch with the finger lightly resting on the scar, but Bella is very body-aware and reported that it "felt like a light touch that burrowed inwards and deep into the abdomen; this got hot and felt like internal tension was being lessened/ was moving. The release and 'pushing out' of the finger felt like a flower inside blooming and unravelling and pushing upwards and outwards and a great sense of relaxation of the structures inside the abdominal cavity." The treatment ended with fascial unwinding of the pelvic transverse diaphragm and an occipital-sacral balance to integrate.	"Range of mobility greatly increased. Ability to stand upright with less pain and walk more evenly and fluidly and move left leg and hip with greatly decreased pain. Range of movement in left leg and hip significantly increased from moving the leg/hip forward/back 5–10 cm with pain to 20–25 cm with minimal pain. Lasting effects: 50%+ decrease in abdomen swelling and size. Opening bowels much easier and less painful. Still difficult but less struggle to get stool out. Shape of stool improved; still flat but no longer ribbon thin. General pain decreased." Bella was also coping better with getting in and out of a car and managing stairs, and had been taking the dog for a walk, which she hadn't done since before the 2017/2018 flare up.
2	FLS for 30 minutes, then DTRH on a laparoscopy scar in the lower left quadrant of abdomen, and finally work was started to the primary scar; now possible as the abdomen was much less reactive. FLS was used under the right ribs where Bella was very tender; this technique appears to be useful in tender and painful areas even where there is no scarring. The abdomen also started to release internal torsion with gentle assistance. Body Realignment was used to free up myofascial patterning created by the internal tension. The approach to Bella's scars was cautious, the concern being to avoid flare-up of symptoms, but she responded well to ScarWork and was nearly blissful at having her much-abused abdomen treated with such a light touch; her joy at what was happening in her body was evident.	"Range of mobility greatly increased. Can stand more upright with less pain, walk more evenly/fluidly with increased speed and stability. Ability to move left leg/hip with greatly decreased pain – ROM increased to 30–45 cm. Lasting effects: Increase in movement gives relief to posture and related pain. Opening bowels easier and less painful again, with constipation beginning to lessen. Burning pain in lower left 'sausage' begins to minimize. Pain lessened with increased movement. General pain again decreased." Two days after the last session Bella had turned to the right and felt as if there was a 'ripping' in the lower left quadrant of the abdomen – the pain went, and she has felt better since; this may be the freeing of adhesions following the session. Managing stairs has been less easy since last treatment, however, due to a discomfort deep in the left hip, which implies further work to the myofascial patterning is required.

continued

Table 11.1 Summary of Bella's treatments and results *continued*

Treatment	Treatment summary	Treatment summary report of result of treatment (obtained during follow-up session)
3	With the aim of helping the left hip shift, the focus was on the laparoscopy scars, lower left quadrant, which gave her a radiating sensation through the body. Work to the internal abdominal torsion was felt deeply by Bella: "Abdominal torsion work & slightly deeper bowel/womb/ovary work: Deep internal pulling and felt very tight but was a very blissful peaceful feeling when it released and it felt good – like tension had been released and it could relax (felt significant due to such a long time of being unable to relax inside)". Body Realignment was then used to positionally release the lumbar area, hips and groin with an occipito-sacral balance to integrate the work.	"Significant improvement in posture, ability to stand straighter without the abdominal 'pulling' I had become so used to. Range of movement increased in abdomen, e.g. could twist without agony – still sensitive and tender but now possible. ROM in legs greatly increased. Walking upright properly, but not yet fully stable. Opening bowels easier and significantly less painful, no strenuous or forceful pushing required (first time in months). Stool still deformed but significantly normalized. Lasting effects: increased ROM retained resulting in more relaxed abdomen and improved posture. Increased ability to do day-to-day tasks more easily with less pain and pulling inside. Increased independence in daily tasks and diversity of tasks. Opening bowels easier again. Burning pain in lower left 'sausage' begins to minimize – still exists but now just flare-ups instead of constant pain; usually linked with obstruction or constipation. General pain again decreased". Bella suffers from crippling period pains which, this month, lasted for two weeks and included bad constipation she feels was induced by a barium transit study. She is gaining weight; has been as low as 47 kg and is now 49 kg.
4	Primary scar worked on and the tissue is now allowing access at a deeper level. This does not mean the therapist is working more deeply, but that the light work is accessing deeper tissues. Matching Layers technique led into more abdominal torsion work and Bella said: "Deep internal pulling and pressure, felt very tight but when it released it felt good – like tension had been released and it could move more freely as a gut should." Direct Fascial Release used to release the platysma, and Sharon Wheeler's BoneWork to the left rib which was protruding abnormally; Bella stated: "The rib did not sit correctly, and once work began, it was a slightly unusual feeling and the rib suddenly dropped down into a more natural position and, although a surprise, this was not uncomfortable or painful. Once the rib had settled into position breathing felt easier and more even and my shoulders felt like they were more balanced and in better alignment and have stayed that way at time of writing."	Bella reported that she is thinking of returning to work part-time; she has not worked since the November 2017 flare-up. For the "first time in years", when her period came this month, she needed no analgesia and experienced no vomiting or fainting. However, she reports having had two reflexology sessions since her last treatment to help a friend who was in training. This is the first time since she started ScarWork treatment and she has agreed to have no further complementary therapy sessions, in order to maintain the accuracy of this case study. Walking is more coordinated, and she reports easier breathing since the ribs were worked on last session. Lasting effects of the July treatment were: "Vibrations in gut and 'baby kicking' sensations minimized and more infrequent instead of constant. Obstructions lessening and sometimes self-resolving; can feel bowel contents force through instead of getting stuck and burning. This helps to minimize the 'sausage' issues and the related pain of constipation and bowel obstructions. Period pain significantly reduced. Into the realms of manageable instead of utterly debilitating. General pain again decreased."

continued

Table 11.1 Summary of Bella's treatments and results *continued*

Treatment	Treatment summary	Treatment summary report of result of treatment (obtained during follow-up session)
5	Laparoscopy scars DTRH, Direct Fascial Release work to ribs and platysma. Right abdominal torsion work. Fascial unwinding of the pelvic diaphragm and left leg. Occipito-sacral balance.	"Large reduction in internal pulling and vibrations, as a result posture has improved; minimized pain when moving. Less feeling of being wrapped up inside, particularly in lower abdomen/hips. Significant reduction in bloat and feeling of being blocked up internally. Ability to move shoulders easier/more fluidly. Bowel feels less angry and less tight; tender and as though it had been handled but not in an unpleasant or uncomfortable way. Ability to process food increased with expansions to the diet being tolerated better with fewer side-effects. The vibrations and feeling of food forcing through the gut minimized again, although not gone completely, the severity of sensation is minimized when they do occur. 4 x transverse colon blocks since August session but used liquid diet to flush it through."
6	FLS to sternum, sub-clavicular area, and around breasts. Laparoscopies and abdominal scar continued. Bella said at the time that: "The work to the breast bone, neck, collar bones and armpits was all very gentle and light and triggered sensations all through the jaw and the face and although an unusual sensation and not one I'd felt before, it was not painful or unpleasant but at times felt warm. Additional sensations of strings/bands pulling/moving in the jaw and face." The feeling of freeness in Bella's chest was significant when standing up after treatment. The release across the chest and shoulders meant that the arms could move backward with much more ease, with none of the associated pulling or pain she had been so used to.	The change in range of motion for the chest and the neck and arms has meant that all walking, sitting, standing, has improved. The lessening of tightness and discomfort has meant the ability to sit at a desk and work has become a real possibility. Bella has bought an automatic car – previously brought to clinic by family members. She can get in and out of a car much more easily and is no longer affected by uneven road surfaces; she is delighted by her new independence.

continued

Table 11.1 Summary of Bella's treatments and results *continued*

Treatment	Treatment summary	Treatment summary report of result of treatment (obtained during follow-up session)
7	On arrival, Bella reports a feeling of tension stemming from the left axilla, across to under right breast, behind to right scapula and down to left sacroiliac joint. All lower abdominal laparoscopy scars worked on with DTRH, but this time it felt as if a very different pattern was being released. While work was being done to the supra-pubic scar, Bella became aware of adhesions to the pubic bone and the connection to the left axilla and right scapula. ScarWork to the abdomen. Body Realignment to clear compensation pattern. Occipito-sacral balance.	"The freedom of movement has remained following the last session and the naturalness of walking has shown the greatest improvement. Stretching arms up and leaning back (not possible without severe internal pulling and accompanied pain prior) is no longer painful, with the intensity of pulling minimized. A previous sensation of pulling under the right rib down to the right hip and pubic bone is greatly reduced and it is much more comfortable to breathe, move and function."
8	More abdominal torsion work to help the deeper adhesions. Bella reported: "This was deep work but pain free. As soon as the tension was found and work began, the body needed it and wanted it. The torsion release gave numerous sensations of peeling, similar to an orange segment being pulled apart and this was a wonderful feeling. Work over the small to large intestine valve was felt deeply as a release of tension in up and down bands from the middle of the R/H side of the abdomen to the pubic bone below." Anterior iliac crests/ASIS restrictions cleared left and right.	Results most notable in the lower left quadrant of the abdomen; the 'sausage' is much less severely painful, and the pain is now above the scar rather than beneath it in the lower left/hip region. "This was the worst point on the abdomen and to have this relieved to this degree is life-changing. Evacuating the bowels is much easier, the narrowings are not there unless wheat is eaten (inflammatory response). This change has been huge for independence and personal progression – hope of a real life back came following the progress of the last session."
9	Work to adhesions within pelvis and Direct Fascial Release to free the pubic bone.	"The ability to stand up straighter without a left/right diagonal pulling is noticeable. The bands that pulled from opposite armpit to hip feel severely lessened and there is a feeling of openness in the bowel, chest, neck, hips. The feeling of balance has improved in my hips and I have a more natural gait when walking. The reduction in abdominal tension was felt immediately and this was as though a muscle cramping had let go but in multiple locations across the abdomen. Subsequent period pain has been greatly improved – an ibruprofen will now suffice for me to live with a dull ache, rather than the life-controlling need to lie down, scream, cry and pass out which I had become accustomed to."

continued

Table 11.1 Summary of Bella's treatments and results *continued*		
Treatment	**Treatment summary**	**Treatment summary report of result of treatment (obtained during follow-up session)**
10	Bella had had four days of severe pain due to a bowel restriction after eating leeks but had managed to pass the stool. She has noticed that, even with an obstruction, the 'sausage' is no longer evident, which she takes as a huge step forward. Abdominal torsion: Deep tension released in/around/under both side of the ribcage. ROM immediately increased and the feeling of being 'matted up' inside was greatly reduced immediately. It felt as if the colon started to unstick from the ribcage/diaphragm areas and the feeling of being kinked inside was greatly lessened.	Bella will continue treatment even though the case study is now finalized.

Bella continues to be very careful with her diet but is optimistic that further improvements will occur, and she is very pleased with how diverse it is now as prior to treatment she had been on clear liquids only for a period of five months.

Bella continues to have treatment and says: "Before finding ScarWork I had reached an impasse in getting help. I had proved very complex and this was causing large delays in practical treatment from the NHS so, unable to continue living in such pain, I tried this treatment with life-altering results. I had, for the previous five months, spent most of my time in bed; even walking to the toilet next door required help. I had lost almost all my independence and had come to accept that my life may never be what I had known. ScarWork has changed my life through minimizing my pain to a point where I am no longer bed-ridden, the number of intestinal obstructions I experience is hugely reduced – this widens the food groups I can now tolerate; I have gained weight and have had tremendous improvement in range of motion; all of this has compounded to give me hope for a brighter future. I am now driving again, have moved into my own flat and am working part-time. Although it's been a difficult two years, the amount of improvement from a non-surgical treatment is astounding and I cannot wait to see where it takes my condition and life next. From the bottom of my heart, thank you!"

References

Tozzi, P. (2014). Fascial Unwinding (Chapter 10, page 147). In Chaitow, L. [editor], Fascial Dysfunction, *Manual Therapy Approaches*. Edinburgh, UK: Handspring Publishing.

INDEX

Note: page numbers followed by b, f, or t indicate a box, figure, or table, respectively

INDEX